The Sensitive Ones

THE SENSITIVE ONES

Healing and Understanding Your Child's Mental Health

Heather Nardi

The Empath Mama

This book details the author's personal experiences with and opinions about mental health. The author is not a trained health-care provider. The statements made about products and services have not been evaluated by the US Food and Drug Administration. They are not intended to diagnose, treat, cure, or prevent any condition or disease. Please consult with your own physician or health-care specialist regarding the suggestions and recommendations made in this book.

Neither the author nor the publisher will be liable for damages arising out of or in connection with the use of this book. You understand that this book is not intended as a substitute for consultation with a licensed health-care practitioner, such as your physician. Before you begin any health-care program or change your lifestyle in any way, you will consult your physician or another licensed health-care practitioner to ensure that you are in good health and that the examples contained in this book will not harm you.

This book provides content related to physical and/or mental health issues. As such, use of this book implies your acceptance of this disclaimer.

ISBN 13: 978-1-63489-484-5

Library of Congress Catalog Number has been applied for.
Printed in the United States of America
First Printing: 2022

26 25 24 23 22   5 4 3 2 1

Cover design by Emily Mahon
Interior design by Patrick Maloney

Wise Ink Creative Publishing
807 Broadway St. NE
Suite 46
Minneapolis, MN 55413

For my supportive spouse, Mario,
and my loving children, Ellie and Lucca.

And to all those that walked alongside
our family during part of this journey.

CONTENTS

DEFINITIONS

Highly Sensitive Person is a term coined by Dr. Elaine Aron. She began researching high sensitivity in 1991 and continues to do research. Dr. Aron's definition of the highly sensitive person (HSP) is "someone that has a sensitive nervous system, is aware of subtleties in his/her surroundings, and is more easily overwhelmed when in a highly stimulating environment."

Empaths, as defined by Dr. Judith Orloff, are "highly sensitive, finely tuned instruments when it comes to emotions. They feel everything, sometimes to an extreme, and are less apt to intellectualize feelings. Intuition is the filter through which they experience the world. Empaths are naturally giving, spiritually attuned, and good listeners. If you want heart, empaths have got it. Through thick and thin, they're there for you, world-class nurturers."

Sensitive Empath is someone who is both a Highly Sensitive Person and Empath.

Empathy, as defined by the Merriam-Webster Dictionary, is "the action of understanding, being aware of, being sensitive to, and vicariously experiencing the feelings, thoughts, and experience of another of either the past or present without having the feelings, thoughts, and experience fully communicated in an objectively explicit manner." Empathy has many levels from a high level to lack of empathy.

Sensitive One is a term I use to define people who feel deeply, who are misunderstood by society, who see life with a different perspective; the creatives, intuitive, with their hearts wide open. We are also known as highly sensitive persons or empaths. This book is titled after you!

INTRODUCTION

> *"The worst loneliness is to not be comfortable with yourself."* —Mark Twain

"Stop trying to fix me," were the words that came out of my ten-year-old daughter's mouth.

I have never forgotten that statement, and I have played it over in my mind many times. At first, I didn't understand. My daughter was two years into her mental health journey, and her therapist had given her tools and new coping skills for her anxiety. I was doing my best to support her, and I thought, how could my child not see that I was trying to be helpful?

As the years went on, I questioned what I was doing to make her feel that way. Never once did I ask her. I think the truth is, I knew it was something I was doing wrong, and I didn't want to hear it. As I healed and accepted truths about myself, I began to understand it was true. I was trying to fix her. I didn't want her to feel the world so profoundly like I do. I thought if I could mold my child into someone else, her life would be easier.

I wasn't accepting the truth of who she is.

Growing up sensitive is not easy. I know, because I am a sensitive empath too. According to Andre Sólo, writing on HighlySensitiveRefuge.com, "Empaths are highly sensitive individuals who are keenly aware of the emotions of those around them, to the point of feeling those emotions themselves." As highly sensitive persons (HSP), we are born with a nervous system that processes experiences and feelings much more deeply than the average person. I didn't know this was who I was until I discovered it for my child.

I knew I was different from most people in my life. I felt emotions intensely, I was a quiet observer, I could feel others' pain when they were hurt, I listened closely when others spoke, and I was the good girl. I got good grades, was never in trouble, and I was polite and friends with everyone.

Every night at dinner, my family would watch the nightly news. While eating, if I saw something disturbing on the screen, I would close my eyes, plug my ears, and leave the dinner table. I couldn't handle the distress I saw on the TV because I was actually feeling it myself. My family never teased me about my behavior; they accepted this as my personality. To me, being sensitive felt weak. It came along with other words to describe me like "shy," "timid," "bashful," and "quiet." I accepted that as my truth for most of my life.

I was what others wanted me to be for them. When you live your life this way, you never really know the authentic you. I was a chameleon changing who I was to fit a situation or another person's needs. This is a common trait for sensitive empaths—we don't want to "rock the boat." We sense others' emotions and give them what they need, even if it means losing ourselves. For my mom, I was the good girl who didn't want to make her upset. For each of my friend groups, I was the friend they needed or wanted. I was a good listener who kept conversations with friends sacred. I was the cheerleader for others when they needed support. I avoided conflict because I wanted to be accepted. I didn't ask for emotional support. If I was struggling, I kept it to myself most of the time.

I went to college because that is what you do after high school. I had a fantastic roommate and made many friends. I didn't always go to class because I felt I could decide if I wanted to go or not. I didn't have anyone watching over me to be the "good girl." It wasn't that I didn't like to learn, but I was nervous around new people and the auditorium-sized classrooms. If I had a friend in my class, I felt comfortable. If not, I felt judged by others, like I didn't fit in my own skin. At the end of freshman year, I was put on probation for the summer because of my poor grades. I returned fall of sophomore year for two quarters, but my experience didn't improve. I was placed on probation again for one year. I never returned. What I know now as a sensitive empath is that I was not prepared to cope with or handle this new environment. I had no awareness of myself and felt lost in the sea of other students.

Since the age of sixteen, I have had a job. I was always a hard worker and a good employee who adapted well to my work environment. I had part-time jobs until I left college and was lucky enough to find a full-time job that led to a career based on my experiences. Around the age of twenty-three, I began to feel more confident in myself.

I met my husband on a blind date when I was twenty-four. I felt a connection with him right away. I felt as if he accepted me, and our relationship quickly became exclusive. After one year together, I found out I was pregnant. We were engaged, married, and living in a house all within five months.

My daughter, Ellie, was a surprise baby. I understand now that she was a gift, and I was supposed to be her parent, but I didn't feel that way in the beginning. I wasn't prepared to have a baby and felt thrown into the path of wife and mother. My entire life flipped from a single working person to a married, stay-at-home mom in just a few short months. To add to all of life's new stresses, Ellie was a challenging baby who became an independent, stubborn toddler with wisdom beyond her years. Someone once told me Ellie was an old soul. I wasn't sure what that meant, but I understand now and I agree. She had a wisdom beyond her years, her vocabulary was expansive, and she was fiercely independent.

As I began to parent Ellie, I unintentionally decided I didn't want her to experience what I had, so I went the other direction by forcing her to be an average child. I didn't want her to feel so deeply or be quiet. I wanted her to fit in and be popular. This is what Ellie meant when she said, "Stop trying to fix me." I realized I was trying to fix her many years later because I didn't want her to struggle. But guess what? She struggled even more because of my desire to change her into someone she wasn't.

Lack of connection with your true voice or sense of self can be a symptom of anxiety. The condition we call "anxiety" has reached staggering numbers in both adults and children. Anxiety will negatively affect your well-being.

I thought Ellie was challenging as a toddler, but then her behavior shifted in third grade to anger outbursts, hitting, kicking, breaking things, verbal attacks, and swearing. All these behaviors were mainly directed toward me. This was the year that changed everything for our family. Most of this behavior occurred when Ellie felt she couldn't control a situation, or something didn't go as she had planned. Many of her outbursts were about attending school.

What surprised me was that she used to love school. She had many friends and was very social. She never missed a day of school, but this all changed in third grade. There were days I would drop her off at school and think, *What would happen if I just kept driving?* Oh, the freedom of going wherever the road would take me, doing what I wanted and not having any responsibility. Moving forward and not looking back. But that is not me. I am a responsible parent who loves her family. At the end of the day, I'd pick Ellie up from school and continue to work through the struggle. It is OK to have these thoughts when we're overwhelmed, but it is how we handle that emotion that predicts the future. If I continued driving, we would have a different story.

Some days I gave in and let her stay home from school because I just didn't have the energy to fight with her. Sometimes I started off strong only to give in after I felt defeat and exhaustion. Then there were the days I totally had it under control; everything was going smoothly, we got to school, and life was good. Those were the days to celebrate, and I thought, *I've got this*, only to have an epic struggle the next day. I never knew what to expect each morning.

I didn't just have one child to raise. I had a son too, and I worked. I was not only a parent but an employee, a member of society, a wife, a friend, and a person in my own right. But I often felt like Ellie controlled me, and I was helpless to do anything but react to her. I lost who I was as a person amid our daily struggles.

I learned to keep this secret from family and friends. I even kept some of my experiences with Ellie quiet from my husband because I felt guilty, and I didn't want to create more stress for him. It is so draining to pretend everything is perfect in your life when at home you feel your child is out of control. If I couldn't handle our eight-year-old daughter, then what kind of parent and wife was I? What would she be like at thirteen, sixteen, or eighteen? Those are the years that are supposed to be challenging for teens and parents. At work, I tried to show up as my happy self, but I felt horrible inside. There were times I would cry on the drive to work, barely able to see the road through my tears. I had to sit in the parking lot and pull myself together before walking through the door. My husband glimpsed the craziness, but mostly it was saved for me.

When Ellie was eight, she received her first diagnosis of generalized anxiety disorder. I walked out of the pediatrician's office with a low-dosage prescription of an antidepressant and a referral for a therapist. I felt a sense of calm, thinking this was the answer to my prayers, the tool that would help with her anxiety.

Even with our most significant attempt to keep our family's secret, it was only a matter of time before our truth was revealed. Ellie's battle with what we thought to be a mental illness was only just beginning. It eventually led to a six-month stay at an inpatient residential treatment facility, where she celebrated her fourteenth birthday. When she returned, we learned that what we thought was a spiral into a profound mental illness was in fact a spiritual awakening with our empathic, sensitive, and intuitive child. When we began alternative treatment options and stopped using prescription medications, we saw an almost immediate shift in our daughter. She is now twenty-one and doing so much better. She has challenging days, but she has tools to cope without spiraling into a dark space.

Living with someone who has a mental illness can be very stressful, making you feel powerless and hopeless, often wanting change. After spending seven years treating Ellie traditionally with therapy, outpatient and inpatient facilities, testing, and prescription medications, we thought, *What are we missing? Why isn't she getting better?*

I felt in my soul there had to be another way. I started to question why children are being diagnosed with mental illness and medicated so young. The increase is staggering, and the list of side effects from prescription medication is long. I was so involved in the mental illness path that I didn't even think to look for another way. It seemed to me her side effects from her prescribed medications were worse than her original diagnosis. Looking back to the start of her mental health care and where we were at this point, a change had to be made to end this cycle. There is a lesson to learn in each moment, and once you accept that change is necessary and befriend this attitude, nothing can disturb your inner peace.

I didn't realize this was the start of a long journey that would teach me to look at mental illness from a different perspective. I didn't realize it was my own healing journey, or that it would lead to my understanding of who my daughter and I are as sensitive empaths.

What if we looked at mental illness differently? Wouldn't you want to understand? Maybe what our children are experiencing are the challenges of being a sensitive or intuitive person. I submerged myself into learning and seeking out information. In this book, I will share what I have learned over the past thirteen years of navigating the journey of mental illness with my child. This is my family's journey, and I don't claim to have medical expertise.

This book has found its way to you and it is meant to be in your hands at this moment in your life. Know this to be true and don't question the why. As you read the words from these pages, know that I hold you in sacred space and send you much love. I have been guided to share my message with those ready to receive it. I hope you will use this book as a resource and share it with those who also need to hear my—and Ellie's—message. The message that with self-understanding comes understanding of others and releasing the need to fix someone else. Understanding is the path to acceptance. Acceptance opened the door to healing, connection, and new perspectives. Once Ellie felt entirely accepted and understood, she could speak up and share what she needed, knowing that I was open to hearing without judgment.

Part One

OUR
JOURNEY

Chapter One

THE EARLY YEARS

W hen I was pregnant with Ellie, I didn't get the typical joy of sharing the news with family. This was not planned, and we weren't married. I felt I was a disappointment to my family for the timing of the pregnancy. My pregnancy was more about the next steps: getting engaged, planning a wedding, getting married, moving into a home with my spouse. I never allowed myself to fully embrace the experience of being pregnant.

I felt disconnected when Ellie was born. I had an emergency C-section and lost a lot of blood. I saw her briefly as they held her up to show me her beautiful face, and then she was swept off with my husband. After hours in recovery, I was brought to a hospital room, and the nurse wheeled her in for me to feed her. I didn't want to feed her. I felt too overwhelmed and exhausted.

There are several studies suggesting that babies are sensitive to their mother's feelings, and even before birth they can absorb the mental and emotional energy of the people around them. Even very young babies are sensitive to the energy of their mothers, absorbing it as part of their development. As a sensitive empathic child ages, these tendencies become more intense. Ellie was sensitive from birth. As an infant, she was easily irritated and would cry. And cry. And cry. Trying to calm her was an exhausting and emotionally wrenching ordeal. As she grew, more of her sensitivities and anxieties emerged; she would get aggressive if something didn't go her way; she had perfectionist behavior and tended to take things personally.

As she got older, she had nightmares and slept with me until she was around six years old. As Ellie grew, we noticed she was knowledgeable; she spoke like an adult with a precise, extensive vocabulary. She enjoyed being around adults and having honest conversations. Ellie had deep, thought-provoking questions, and she worried about occurrences in the world.

Ellie was challenging and complex—or as we liked to call her, spirited. Her bold behavior resulted in constant power struggles as she tested the limits of what we would allow. When she was three, my friend Mickie was over for a visit. Ellie talked with us, got upset about something, stormed off, and slammed her bedroom door. I remember Mickie making a comment about Ellie's behavior, how we would have our hands full when she grew to be a teenager. I let Ellie storm off and express herself. I didn't discipline her for that behavior. Right or wrong, that is how I dealt with Ellie in our home. I was raised in an environment without many rules, but that flexibility worked for me. I was an only child until twelve, and I was a very "good" kid, so that was how I went into parenting my child.

Being Ellie's mom often made me feel tired and defeated. I wondered why she wasn't like other kids, who enjoyed extracurricular activities with ease or listened to their parents while shopping. I had to force Ellie into activities, which caused stress and usually an emotional breakdown from both of us. One time I had her enrolled in a class at the YMCA. I had her convinced to attend but as soon as we walked into the gym for the class she ran to the bathroom and locked the stall door. I stood outside the door trying to convince my daughter to participate in this class. It then turned into frustration, raising my voice, then negotiations. If I said "no" to Ellie in a store, it turned into a barter situation, in which she would not back down until she received the answer she wanted. Was this my parenting, or her personality? Or was it something else?

Ellie never slept well, not even as a baby. She needed lots of comforting, which I tried to provide. I rocked her while listening to music, I sang, I sat on the couch watching TV while holding her, I walked the halls. A friend told me about sleep training for infants where you let the baby cry it out. Nothing seemed to work for Ellie or me. I could not stand to let her cry herself to sleep. It was too much for me to handle. I often felt I was doing everything wrong as a parent. I sought help in parenting books, only to end up feeling worse. The recommendations I found didn't work for my child. This is one example of how different it is to parent an empath or sensitive child as an empath. She probably needed complete silence and not to be overstimulated with sound or movement for her to sleep. She also sensed my frustration of not getting her to sleep, and so the pattern continued over and over.

Friends and family gave advice, trying to be helpful, but I still felt alone and lost. My husband supported me the best he could by offering encouraging words or advice. He took shifts of walking the hall, trying to get our daughter to sleep so his wife could have a moment of peace. I was the parent in the trenches dealing with the everyday challenges. There were nights I would lie in bed crying, not wanting to be a mom anymore. This was not how I imagined having a baby. I guess Ellie could sense my angst. I loved her, but I was struggling.

I think many parents do this, especially first-time parents. We feel we don't have the answers or experience to help our child. Parents envision a fantastic future for our kids, where they are healthy, happy, and successful. When we start to see our child struggling, we look for understanding, which can turn to blame or guilt. Maybe that blame falls on another person, situation, or yourself.

But this reproach reflects your own unrealistic expectations. I remember blaming myself for Ellie's diagnosis. I caused her to be an anxious child, I thought. The list went on: I was a terrible parent, anxiety was in my family's history, etc. But blame doesn't accomplish or change anything. I wasn't in the blame for very long, as I am a very positive person, and I knew it wouldn't achieve anything. I was able to shift my perspective to believe I could learn a lesson through our experience. Little did I know how large the lesson would become.

DIAGNOSED MENTAL ILLNESS

The biggest challenge started in third grade when Ellie was eight years old. One of her main issues was school avoidance. Ellie attended a private school with a small class size. She had many friends, and for the first few years, she was the child that didn't miss a day of school and loved her teachers. So I knew something was wrong when she started fighting me about going to school.

Other signs of her anxiety were excessive worry, fear with no discernible cause, stomachaches, not wanting to participate in outside activities, aggression (mainly toward me), and perfectionism. Ellie became violent if something didn't go as planned or if she didn't have control over a situation. I remember one time we were going to visit my parents for the day and Ellie didn't want to go. She was hitting me, calling me names, and swearing. She took my Kindle from the kitchen table and went into her room. I heard a crash on the floor. A moment later, she walked out of her room with the Kindle in her hand, the screen cracked. I was so upset I couldn't even look her in the eye. I left the house by myself and drove to my parents' house. My husband ended up coming later with both kids, and Ellie apologized.

I kept most of my experiences with Ellie a secret, only giving a few people a glimpse into my real life. Our son was only two years old, and I was worried about what he saw in our house. I took on the responsibility of not sharing to keep others happy and safe. When you live like this, you need to seek out help; this is more than a challenging child. I felt like I was living a lie, and it was a lonely place. My husband and I eventually made the decision that Ellie should see her pediatrician to get to the root of her behavior. I remember that first appointment like it was yesterday. I shared with the doctor my concerns as Ellie sat at the table, not saying a word. Occasionally, she would give me an angry glare. She didn't like me talking about her, especially sharing some of our stories which until now had been kept secret. The doctor asked Ellie questions, and her response was usually, "I don't know," or a shoulder shrug.

I was given the GAD-7 screening tool[1] with seven questions, and asked to rate my answer from zero to three, with zero being "not at all," and three being "nearly every day." I filled it out, knowing the answers I provided were likely showing issues that needed to be resolved.

1. Feeling nervous, anxious, or on edge
2. Not being able to stop or control worrying
3. Worrying too much about different things
4. Trouble relaxing
5. Being so restless that it is hard to sit still
6. Becoming easily annoyed or irritable
7. Feeling afraid as if something awful might happen

From our discussion and questionnaire results, Ellie received her first diagnosis of generalized anxiety disorder. It was recommended that she begin to take a low dosage of a prescription medication called fluoxetine and see a therapist to learn coping skills. Fluoxetine, otherwise known as Prozac, increases levels of a chemical called serotonin in the brain. I was told it would improve Ellie's mood and decrease fear, anxiety, and unwanted thoughts. The doctor also told us the prescription was safe for children and had minimal side effects like headaches, sleep issues, and dry mouth.

To be honest, I was relieved to be given a name for Ellie's behavior and a prescription to help her feel better. My husband wasn't on board with the idea of putting our child on medication.

He didn't even take Tylenol for a headache. On the other hand, I grew up looking to the doctor as the expert, seeking out their expertise often, and using medicine to make me better. I trusted the doctor's information, and was able to convince my husband that medication would be the best plan for our child.

Along with the prescription, the doctor recommended that she see a therapist. We found one near our home, and Ellie enjoyed their time together. She colored and played games while they talked about feelings and skills. The therapist gave me handouts and shared what was discussed or what coping skills Ellie should be practicing at home. For a few days after their session, Ellie felt motivated to work through any behavior issues or use coping skills when feeling anxious. Still, that eagerness faded over the weeks until her next appointment. Ellie didn't like us to remind her of the coping skills she was supposed to be using at home. If we called attention to her behavior in any way, she would get angry.

The combination of therapy and a low dose of antidepressants seemed to help a little. But our daily struggle continued. Life didn't get much better after Ellie's diagnosis. We wanted an end to morning arguments about school, feeling bullied by our own child, fighting over homework in the evening, and living a life on the roller coaster of chaos. We were waiting for that moment when our child would be "normal."

About a year after starting her medication, Ellie was also experiencing migraines, stomach pains, and weight gain. We wondered if these were side effects or something more serious. The migraines were so bad that in fourth grade, she was referred to a neurologist. He requested she have a CAT scan and prescribed a preventative migraine medication to be taken daily.

Around the age of ten, Ellie received a neuropsychological evaluation because we weren't seeing much improvement in her initial diagnosis of generalized anxiety disorder. Neuropsychological testing examines your child's mental abilities as they relate to neurologic or other medical disorders, mental health difficulties, or problems at school. From that testing, we received additional diagnoses: ADHD inattentive type and oppositional defiant disorder.

For our concerns about Ellie's weight gain, we were referred to an endocrinologist, who determined that Ellie had hypothyroidism. Hypothyroidism is an underactive thyroid gland. This means the thyroid gland can't make enough hormones to keep the body running normally.

Brain chemical alterations by a thyroid disorder also impact ADHD symptoms. When you have hypothyroid and ADHD, your body is not sending enough neurotransmitters or processing the right hormones for proper metabolism. This means you may suffer cloudy thinking, low blood pressure, extreme lack of short-term and working memory, and possibly depression. The lack of motivation is often highly frustrating for someone with both disorders. Both ADHD and thyroid disorders delay human functions and influence the ability to succeed socially, at work, school, and more.

With this new diagnosis, I was ready for a plan of action and felt this would give us a better understanding of why Ellie was struggling at school. She was kept on the same prescription medications, and referred to a neuropsychologist instead of a therapist.

But again, my hope to see change was extinguished. Ellie was given coping skills, but she hardly used them, and I couldn't blame her for it.

She was taught different breathing techniques; she could bring a small object like a stone to hold in her hand for comfort; she was told she could leave the classroom and walk around or get a drink of water. But like most children, Ellie didn't want to be different from the other kids or bring attention to herself, so there was no way she was going to get up and leave the classroom. In fifth grade, she jumped off a snowbank and hurt her foot. She didn't want to tell a teacher or the parent on recess duty how hurt she was. She could hardly walk back into the building when recess was over.

One of her friends told the teacher how hurt Ellie was, and the teacher approached her. Ellie told the teacher she was OK. When I picked her up from school, she was limping to the car. Once out of others' eyes, she began to cry and explain how much pain she was in. We went to the urgent care and found out she had a fracture in her foot.

From her neuropsychic appointments, we did see Ellie bring home a lot of coloring sheets, as that is what she spent most of the one-hour session doing. I do believe coloring helped her feel calm during her appointments. She also had someone else to talk to and share her feelings with.

But Ellie was still avoiding school, and she was developing issues with her friends. If someone upset her in any way, she held a grudge and would not forgive them. If she had a late assignment from missing so much school, she wouldn't want to go. We felt like we were in a crazy cycle. At this point, our school was aware of Ellie's mental illness diagnosis and was trying to work with us. Her school principal told us to get her into the building no matter what, even if I had to bring her to the office kicking and screaming. He would take it from there. I tried to get her in the car forcibly, but I often gave up and let her be home. It was too hard for me emotionally.

By this point, Ellie knew how to play the game. She gave the answers the therapist or psychologist was seeking just to get through the appointment. And she remained uncooperative at home.

Chapter Two

THE TEENAGE YEARS

As we moved into Ellie's teenage years, our lives increasingly revolved around her many appointments and unpredictable behavior. In seventh grade, she started at a new public school.

She began to see a school therapist once a week who helped her with any struggles that came up at home or school. She was to be an ally for Ellie.

Being a twelve-year-old girl with anxiety in a new school was too much for Ellie to handle. The school was larger and full of people she didn't know. She felt overwhelmed and lost. Her friends were making new friends, and on several occasions, she was bullied.

In one situation, a group of boys made an inappropriate sexual comment to Ellie as she walked to the bus. Ellie came home in tears.

I went to the school therapist the very next day and shared with her what Ellie had experienced. I felt confident she would understand Ellie, and something would be done about the situation.

"These boys hurt my child," I told her. "She came home emotionally distraught by their words and intentions as she was walking to the bus after school."

I wanted action from the therapist, but I was told, "We define bullying as any physical, verbal, or psychological abuse among schoolchildren that occurs repeatedly over a period of time. Those boys shouldn't have said what they did to Ellie, but it doesn't fall under our definition of bullying."

"Besides," the therapist continued, "Ellie dishes it out as much as she takes it."

I couldn't believe what I was hearing. This was Ellie's "ally," the person who was supposed to be in her corner. We tell our children from a young age to "tell a trusted adult if you are experiencing bullying." That is exactly what Ellie did and there was no action step to move forward.

I didn't get validation for my child's experience. I was shut down by the therapist.

Anger boiled through me as I walked out of that office, past the "No Bullying" sign, which seemed to taunt me from its place on the wall. It didn't feel like a safe space for my child. Ellie was afraid to attend school, and yet that didn't qualify as bullying.

A few days later, still infuriated, I searched the internet for information on bullying. I stumbled upon a local organization called Pacer Center. I reached out to them and shared Ellie's story. They provided a sympathetic ear, and also offered a variety of options on how to approach the school principal or school board. Ellie didn't want me to share this situation with anyone else. She didn't want the attention or to share the names of the students who made those comments to her. Because Ellie was so sensitive to emotions, the school building itself became a trigger for her. Going near it made her replay what happened during that school year, and the emotions of the other students were too much for her.

Ellie started to withdraw, and began fighting me about going to school again. One day, while I was driving her to school because she missed the bus, she threatened to jump out of the moving car. I didn't want to think she would do it, but I could see this happening. In my mind's eye, I could see Ellie putting her hand on the door handle, opening the door, and rolling out onto the road. The thought terrified me. I pushed the lock button on the door again and again, watching her in the rearview mirror until I could turn the car around and take her home. My stomach was a pit of hopelessness. My daughter would rather have jumped out of a moving car than go to school. No parent wants this for their child.

Shortly before this happened, we made a shift, per the school therapist, to see a colleague of hers for prescription medication management. It was a psychiatrist from the same office as Ellie's therapist. We didn't realize at the time how much of a connection existed between Ellie's behavior and her shifts in medication. But we soon came to understand her behavior changed when she switched from Prozac to Cymbalta. She had been on her other medicines for an extended period without much change, and the new psychiatrist thought the difference would be suitable for her chemically as she grew older. This felt like the next transition in Ellie's mental health care, and again, I followed the doctor's recommendation. Looking back, I feel like the Cymbalta brought on new symptoms that she didn't experience before, like depression and suicidal ideation.

Ellie's school avoidance became a huge issue in seventh grade. While we had more flexibility and acceptance in our private school, public schools have a strict attendance policy. Ellie struggled with the transition into this new school, and her newly adjusted meds caused symptoms we didn't expect. The school threatened us with truancy, and said we could be taken to court for our child not attending school. The school therapist was working with the school truancy officer regarding Ellie's attendance issues. The therapist explained the situation with Ellie's mental illness to the truancy officer at the school, but this was not enough to stop him from reaching out to my husband and me and asking for a meeting.

"It is against the law for a child not to be in school and receive an education," he told Ellie. "And if you don't start coming to school regularly, your parents could be taken to court for neglect."

The truancy officer said I should call my local nonemergency police to come to pick up my daughter and bring her to school if I could not get her on the bus or in the car myself. Call the police to bring an anxious and depressed teen to school! *What?* This didn't feel right to me! There was no way I would call a police officer to force my child into a police car for school. I knew this would cause more trauma. I couldn't imagine how my child would feel having to step out of the car with a police officer at her school. She was being treated like a criminal.

All this pressure from the school combined with my daily struggles as a parent to a child with mental illness was overwhelming. I couldn't focus and all my days blended together. Then I got a phone call to schedule a home visit from a county caseworker. I thought, *Now what?* We were in the space of intervention. An unsolicited outsider was coming into our home to evaluate our daughter's well-being.

The caseworker came to meet with me as my husband could not get off work. She introduced herself, took out her notebook and pen, and started asking questions. I'd been answering similar questions since third grade when we started this journey with Ellie. For about an hour, the caseworker listened to my responses to her questions and wrote in her notebook.

As the end of the appointment drew near, she set down her pen and looked at me. "I think what your daughter is experiencing is due to parenting," she said. She went on to share how Ellie needed strict discipline and boundaries. I was so surprised and taken aback that I sat there and listened without responding. I think I even thanked her for coming.

The moment the door closed behind her, I began to sob. I was so confused. If our parenting was the culprit, didn't she think we would have resolved our issues years ago before putting our child on medications and driving her to endless appointments? I called my husband at work and told him what happened. He could tell I was overwhelmed, and spoke calmly.

"She probably had to share another perspective on Ellie's case," he said, and advised me not to take it personally.

But how could it be anything but personal? Maybe I wasn't the best parent, and I could have done some things differently. As I write this, years later, I feel a range of emotions. No parent should have to be told their parenting is to blame when their child is threatening to harm themselves and won't even leave their room. I often felt I was the primary decision-maker, an emotional punching bag and always present in Ellie's battle.

We made a combined decision with the school and Ellie's therapist that Ellie would end seventh grade two weeks early since she wasn't attending anyway. As a condition, we had to register her for a partial hospitalization program for the summer. We agreed and moved forward feeling like we put an end to that year.

Ellie began to attend the partial hospitalization program the summer before eighth grade. I dropped her off and picked her up after seven hours of group sessions, and both private and family therapy. She participated willingly for a couple of days, but soon we were back to the same struggles we had with school. I couldn't get her into the car or even out of bed. Threats of punishment didn't matter to Ellie. She didn't care about anything; she hated life and people. This program reminded her of school, and she felt judged by others in the program.

If we couldn't get her to attend, her team told us they would recommend Ellie be sent to an inpatient hospitalization program, where they could do symptom stabilization while adjusting her medications. I felt like we were punishing our child for not attending a program by locking her in a different program. We sat Ellie down to explain the importance of attending the day program and the consequences if she continued missing days. But the threat didn't sink in.

"I don't care," said Ellie. She didn't believe there would be consequences for her behavior because we as parents didn't often follow through with our punishment threats.

One of the worst days of my life was the day we had to take

action on Ellie's behavior. Even though I didn't totally agree with the decision, I went along with the professionals. I woke up that morning knowing Ellie was going to be transported to an inpatient hospitalization program. I couldn't tell her or she wouldn't get in the car with me. I pretended we had a routine visit with her therapist at the program that morning. With my stomach tied in a knot, I dropped off my son at daycare, and with Ellie by my side, I drove, not really knowing what to expect and trying to pretend it was a typical day.

We parked the car and started to walk in. Ellie sensed something was off; she was hesitant to go with me. I reaffirmed that we were attending an appointment. We checked in at the front desk, and were waved upstairs to the program area. Each step I took felt like I was stepping through mud. When we reached the top of the stairs, Ellie definitely started to sense something was not right. I could see it in her eyes. A staff member was waiting for us and noticed Ellie's demeanor. At that point, Ellie turned and tried to leave, a code was called, and other staff members surrounded her.

"I hate you!" she yelled to me.

My heart broke into pieces as I responded, "I love you."

Staff directed me to an empty office by the entrance while they prepared Ellie for transport. I called my husband at work to let him know what was happening. I sat alone peeking from the door as I watched my daughter tied down on a stretcher, being carted away to the ambulance. Tears flowed down my face, and I felt despair and heartbreak like never before. How did this happen to our family?

In a room all alone, Ellie would stay overnight with no doors on her bathroom, and only certain items allowed in her room for her own safety. For five days, we visited her every evening until her release. She attended programming individually and with peers, but no medications were adjusted. At the end of her stay, they recommended that Ellie continue the partial hospitalization program, the one she struggled to participate in. I guess they believed she was magically ready to go back to the original plan after five days of treatment in a locked facility without family.

We didn't feel like anything was accomplished from her time at this facility except for Ellie feeling punished. My husband and I discussed what we believed would be best for Ellie. We thought having her home and spending time with family and friends would be more inspiring than going back to the program. So, against the doctor's orders, we pulled Ellie out of all programs with this facility. For the first time, we listened inwardly to what we thought was best for our child, but it upset the system and her doctors. When I told the doctor at the facility about our plans, she called my husband at work to confirm. This was fine as we were both in agreement, but I guess she didn't believe me! She asked that my husband sign paperwork confirming that we pulled our child out against the doctor's order.

We spent the last month of summer just being and not trying to force Ellie into any programs. Ellie spent time with friends and family. There was a sense of peace and calm in our home. We felt like a "normal" family, laughing and spending time together. Ellie was getting excited for the start of eighth grade. We had big hopes for a fresh start with seventh grade behind us. Well, that feeling changed quickly.

On the first day of school, Ellie was hesitant to go to the bus stop at the top of our street. I finally convinced her to start walking. She got about halfway before she turned around and came home, refusing to go to school. She missed the first day of eighth grade.

This was the start of our worst year. Ellie only attended school for a few weeks, as she started to spend more time in her room, secluding herself from family and friends. My daughter, who had once been a social butterfly, would lie in her bed with the covers over her head, saying she hated life. She didn't want come out of her room to eat, so I brought her food. Some of her close friends came to our door asking to talk with her, but she didn't want to see them. You could tell by their faces that her friends were so concerned for Ellie, but they also seemed confused and didn't understand what she was experiencing. I chatted with them for a few minutes and thanked them for coming. I missed seeing Ellie with her friends. I missed having a child who attended school and was a part of life. As the weeks passed, the visits to our door became fewer and fewer until there were no more.

I had heard of depression on TV and the radio. I learned symptoms of depression in high school and college health class, but I was now experiencing it firsthand with my child. Depression symptoms aren't always as apparent as frequent crying and overwhelming despair. Often the changes are subtle and happen over time, which can make it difficult to notice. In our house, depression came along like a dark cloud we didn't see moving overhead until it was directly upon us.

Ellie spent all her time in her bed; she still struggled to sleep. I was genuinely concerned that she'd withdrawn from friends and her everyday activities. She wouldn't even go out to dinner with family, which she usually loved to do. As her mom, I could see her eyes were dark, and my daughter was no longer there. She hated life, she hated people, and all she wanted to do was sleep and play on the computer.

Since Ellie wouldn't leave our home and wasn't getting better without support, we had a therapist come into our house. This didn't seem to help. Ellie would maybe come out of her room to see the therapist and if she did, she might answer a question with "I don't know," or "I don't care," or a shoulder shrug. The therapist even brought up the idea that maybe Ellie was on the autism spectrum because my depressed daughter wouldn't make eye contact or be social. I felt as if we received a new diagnosis each time she saw a different therapist or doctor. We were all doing the best we could for her care, but working with mental illness symptoms could still be frustrating for everyone involved.

Ellie was experiencing suicidal thoughts. When asking her a question or trying to have a conversation, she would often respond, "I wish I was dead," or "You probably wish I was dead." One day, I opened her bedroom door to find her sitting on her bed with a pair of scissors and chunks of her hair in a pile. I reacted calmly so I didn't startle her. She couldn't explain to me what she was doing or why. I was afraid this was the beginning of self-harm. I cleaned it up and told her we could go to our hairstylist and have her hair evened out. I didn't know the right way to respond, but I did feel freaking out would cause her to react in the same way. Being calm seemed to be the best approach with Ellie.

Once, when she was upset about something, Ellie reached for a kitchen knife. For a moment, I wondered if she would use the knife to harm me. I was afraid of my own child. I stood in front of her and the knife block in the corner of the kitchen, and calmed her down by holding her arms against her body and talking slowly. Moments later, she apologized. I had seen this behavior before. She would appear to be in a trance and not fully aware of what she was saying or doing out of anger or sadness. Then she would come back and feel horrible for what she did and apologize.

I feared leaving her alone in the house because it would only take one moment of not thinking clearly to end her life. I would probably have been the one to find her, so I prepared myself in some weird way that this could happen. I tried to walk in the house first, go into her room, crack open the door calling her name, and hope for a response. No parent should feel that way. I had to come to the point where I surrendered to what might happen. I couldn't let the what-ifs or maybes control my everyday feelings. I still had my own life to continue.

I felt as if Ellie's in-home therapist was more for me. Since Ellie would not come out to participate and we were paying for the time, I shared with her the situations we were experiencing as a family. She recommended we keep all medications in a lockbox and put away knives or other items that could be used for harm. She brought up the idea of sending Ellie to an inpatient residential treatment facility.

"When your child has a broken arm," she said, "you take her to the doctor. Since your child is struggling and won't leave her room, she needs care outside of the home." When she explained it to me in that way, I understood. Ellie was not getting better or even trying to get better. She was not participating in life.

My husband and I came to the gut-wrenching decision to send our daughter to an inpatient residential treatment facility eighty miles from our home, following the recommendation of our in-home therapist. This was a decision we had to make for the best interest of our family. This is the decision I hoped I would never have to make. The time between making the decision and driving Ellie to the facility was the longest four weeks of my life. It was right before Christmas, and we decided to wait until January to admit her. We didn't want her to be away from family for Christmas. For safety reasons, we didn't tell her about the upcoming stay. We weren't sure if that would put her over the edge to harm herself, hurt one of us, or run away.

The night before we left for our long drive to the facility, I packed up things she could bring with her, some photos of friends and family, and I wrote a note.

Dear Ellie, it began. *We love you so much . . .*

I put everything in the trunk. The following day, Ellie thought she had an appointment with a new doctor. We lied to our child once again because we thought she might jump out of the moving car, run away, or harm someone. We knew she would fight this decision and not go freely.

The whole drive, I felt uneasy and emotional. We were carrying on a normal conversation with her so she wouldn't pick up on anything. We parked the car right out front and entered the building. She walked in with us but as soon as she felt something was not right about the situation, she turned toward the front door and ran. She was like an animal being hunted. She bolted down a steep snowbank with her father chasing after her. I asked the front desk person for help.

She responded, "We can't help because she is not officially a patient."

I walked outside, searching for my daughter and husband in the cold January weather, and saw the two of them slowly walking toward me. Their legs were covered with snow, their cheeks red and their hands cold. Ellie was crying. I tried to comfort her, but she was angry. Angry at parents who lied to her again, angry that she was somewhere unknown, angry at life.

We met a staff member in the lobby and followed her to an office space, where we began the process of admitting our daughter. The three of us met with various people at the facility. It was an old orphanage with four two-story brick homes, a chapel, and a central space for meeting. It felt like a college campus, but Ellie was not there for education—she was there for mental health services. We talked with the therapist who would be working directly with Ellie. She was friendly and helpful in comforting her.

"We will be meeting tomorrow, Ellie," said the therapist, "and we'll talk more then." Then Ellie had a chance to see her room and meet her roommate. She was surprised to see some of her personal items on the bed in the room. I told her to let me know what other items I should bring next time we saw her.

Before long, it was time for her dad and me to leave. We were leaving our child with strangers, and we had to trust they would provide her the best care. The pain in my heart was pure anguish, but I held it together for my daughter and husband. We hugged Ellie and I whispered in her ear, "I love you."

"I love you, too," she responded. Her dad gave her a hug and we walked out of the building to our car. I was holding back tears and had a lump in my throat. In the car, my husband began to cry. I had never seen him cry before, not even when his father passed. It was like all the years and all our struggles had culminated into this moment. I gave him space to release his feelings, and listened to and acknowledged his emotions. Once we both felt settled, we drove off knowing we would be back to visit soon. Ellie spent her fourteenth birthday and six months of her life at this inpatient residential facility, away from her family and friends. By the time she came home, our lives would change again, but not in the way we thought.

Chapter Three

GROWING UP SENSITIVE

Parenting was different during my childhood. My mom stayed at home with me, which she felt pressured to do, and she reminded me of that often. We lived in the suburbs with many kids in the neighborhood. I was an only child until my brother, a surprise baby, came along when I was twelve. I don't recall my mom playing with me or helping with homework. I spent most of my time outside with the neighbors. There weren't many rules or boundaries in our home and that seemed to work for me.

My parents occasionally expressed their love verbally or with affection, but more by providing my needs like food, clothes, gifts, and privileges. As a sensitive child, I craved deep emotional connections and validation. I knew I was different, and I wanted someone to say that was OK.

I learned to keep my emotions to myself and not upset others. I never knew how my mom would react to a situation or behavior. One moment she could seem happy and the next be yelling and slamming doors. This was particularly challenging for me as a sensitive child who took on the emotions of others. I felt as if I was walking on eggshells most of my childhood. I knew my mother loved me, but I didn't want to be the cause of her upset or disappointment. This was true with most of my relationships.

I recall when I was at our family's cabin, and we were returning from a boat ride. I was probably about five years old. My great-uncle and I both got off the boat at once, and my toe was smashed between the boat and the dock. Instead of saying anything or making a sound, I walked toward my mom and started to cry. I didn't want my great-uncle to feel bad for hurting me. Taking on pain rather than letting others know they hurt me has been a common reaction throughout my life.

For a long time, I didn't think I had a voice that anyone would hear. As a child, I was called shy, timid, reserved, and bashful. As a teen, I heard the words snobbish or stuck up from others to describe my personality. These words are often used to describe someone who is quiet or keeps to themselves, but they were upsetting because they seemed hurtful and carried a negative connotation. I didn't feel people knew the real me. I was caring, funny, and a good friend, but I felt I wasn't worthy of sharing or speaking my thoughts. I was also called "smiley" because I always had a smile on my face. I was trying to project a happy person to everyone even though I felt misunderstood underneath that smile. The smile was my way of approaching the world positively.

As someone quiet, I also was a keen observer and a great listener. I was very aware of my surroundings, listened to everyone, and took in what they were saying. When entering a room, it was as if I had my antenna up and perceived at a high level all of what was going on around me. I could also sense what others felt, causing me to feel anxiety and worry.

With shyness, my deepest fears were rejection and judgment. I worried when I did speak, it would not be well received or understood. In elementary school, I remember a boy teasing me about the sound of my voice when I read aloud in class; he said it was quiet and high-pitched. That caused me to go even more inward. In college, I didn't even like to use the phone to order pizza. I would ask my friends to do it for me. I felt sick to my stomach when having to share my talk in speech class. I avoided a speech in my English class in college and failed the course, which led to me being on probation for my grades. Not having an awareness of who I truly was as a person kept me from opportunities out of my fear of judgment during those years.

I started to use food and external things to fill me up. I wanted to appear perfect to others even though I felt lost inside. This food issue started around seventh grade and continued well into my adulthood. My weight increased in college, more like the freshman fifty than the freshman fifteen. To replace my low self-esteem, I had a red sports car, name-brand clothes, and many friends.

When I had my daughter, I didn't want her to feel disappointed. I would often fix situations for her or jump in to resolve an issue. I believe this caused her the inability to regulate her emotions and created a codependent relationship between us. We were intertwined in our feelings. Ultimately, I built a clear sense of, "I'm not OK unless you're OK." This was not teaching good boundaries or healthy limits with my child. Being a sensitive empath and raising an empath (which I didn't know at the time) was difficult for me. I was easily overwhelmed by Ellie's emotions. To feel calm, I would give in to a situation or solve a problem for her.

Ellie was in full-time kindergarten, meaning she went all day for five days a week. There was a half-day option, but I was still working part-time and pregnant with my son, so this was the best option at the time. I worked three days a week, and Ellie knew I was home on certain days. She would ask me if she could attend a half-day and spend the rest of the time with me. I often gave in and picked her up early instead of making her stay for the committed amount of time.

Ellie didn't speak up at school but didn't have that problem at home. She felt comfortable enough to share her true feelings with me. When we attended a conference for Ellie in kindergarten, her teacher said Ellie wouldn't ask her any questions but would send one of her friends to ask for her. We laughed because Ellie had a "crew" that spoke up for her.

It took me a long time to get comfortable with people, but I opened up and became more comfortable with myself once I did. I struggled to approach others I saw as authorities. I was always polite and respectful. This is what I saw in Ellie, too. She was silly and fun with her friends, and quiet and reserved with adults. I think this came from a lack of self-worth and a fear of speaking or acting incorrectly. This fear of authority on my part carried through in the care of Ellie's mental health. I listened to medical professionals and followed their direction without question, and wanted them to perceive me as a good parent.

IS BEING A HIGHLY SENSITIVE PERSON OR EMPATH HEREDITARY?

I couldn't find much scientific evidence or sources to give me an exact answer to this question.

Dr. Elayne Daniels explains, "The Highly Sensitive Person (HSP) is born with the genetic trait of high sensitivity (HS), also known as Sensory Processing Sensitivity. In the 1990's, Dr Elaine Aron wrote a book about the Highly Sensitive Person and popularized the term highly sensitive."[2]

Dr. Judith Orloff, author of *The Empath's Survival Guide*, explains that there are four main factors that can contribute to heightening one's sensitivities. One is genetics. The others are temperament, trauma, and support.[3]

I believe both my parents to be sensitive, but it shows up in different ways. This is the same with my children. My son is sensitive but not to the same high degree as Ellie.

My mom had a father who was physically and emotionally abusive. By the stories I have been told about him, I believe he was a narcissist. Narcissism is a mental condition by which people have, according to MayoClinic.org, "an inflated sense of their own importance, a deep need for excessive attention and admiration, troubled relationships, and a lack of empathy for others." Narcissists are often attracted to highly sensitive people or empaths because they naturally have a giving nature and narcissists thrive on the need to feel important. I believe my grandmother was sensitive, and he was attracted to her partly because of that trait. I never met my grandfather, as my grandparents divorced before I was born, and my mom didn't want any contact with him.

My great-grandmother was institutionalized for having a "nervous breakdown" after the birth of her fourth child. That term was used to describe many types of mental health issues during that era. I wonder if she was sensitive and experiencing an overload in emotion that she couldn't explain. When we live in a high-sensitivity state, it comes with challenges, such as becoming easily overwhelmed, overstimulated, or exhausted, or absorbing stress and negativity from others. Often, this may show up as a mental health crisis.

My mom is sensitive and her dad was a narcissist, so she grew up in a family with a lot of emotional repression. Growing up, I watched my mother struggle with aspects of the childhood trauma she had experienced from her father. As an adult she would become overreactive and lash out easily at times, and those emotions would quickly turn to resentment.

My dad is a sensitive, generous person who comes from a line of others like him. He cries at movies and is easily moved by emotions. He treats all people with kindness and respect. He has always had a positive attitude, and I have rarely seen him angry. I am not sure if he is a highly sensitive person or just a loving, empathic person.

I also believe my children are sensitive in different ways. My daughter is a sensitive empath and my son is a highly sensitive child. These are two different degrees of feeling emotion. Sensitive empaths take the experience of the highly sensitive person much further.

HOW DO WE ACCEPT OUR PAST GENERATIONS AND HEAL TO MOVE FORWARD FOR OUR FUTURE?

Generational trauma is exactly what it sounds like: trauma that isn't just experienced by one person but extends from one generation to the next. "It can be silent, covert, and undefined, surfacing through nuances and inadvertently taught or implied throughout someone's life from an early age onward," licensed clinical psychologist and parenting evaluator Melanie English, PhD, tells *Health*.

From the death of a family member to an abusive relationship, terrible experiences can have a lasting impact on current and future generations.

It's in our nature to be driven by our family histories. They give us invisible threads that tie us to the past. Our past influences us, inspires us, and sometimes holds us back. Our family has some of those experiences. I know my parents wanted a better life for me, but they didn't realize the scars of their own childhood traumas could still cause pain and affect their parenting.

Most parents, including mine, are trying their best. Few have been taught much about raising kids beyond their own experience with their parents. My family had to learn the hard way that what we don't heal, we repeat. I am trying to put a stop to that cycle.

The feeling of being misunderstood and my lack of self-acceptance filtered through my maternal side and continued through Ellie and me. The only way to end it was by healing myself. There are many unique forms of therapy and professionals to help families through generational trauma. The primary way is through knowledge and awareness of our past and current situation. We owe it to our loved ones to break the cycle of trauma. Not everything we inherit is worth passing to our children.

Chapter Four

THE AWAKENING

E llie's first diagnosis at the age of eight years old gave me the role of parent to a child with mental illness. I moved forward without questioning another way. This was our life until I came to a point where I could no longer accept this as our truth. This was my awakening! A spiritual journey ensuing from an awakening is not a planned experience. For me, it came during a dramatic event: bringing my daughter to an inpatient residential treatment facility for mental illness.

My process through awakening started as an awareness. While Ellie was away receiving treatment, I searched for answers about other treatments for mental illness. I needed to find a solution, but I didn't expect the search to lead me down a path of self-discovery. I began to understand myself better and cultivated a different perspective of my role in Ellie's struggles with mental illness. I read books on self-love and attended classes on meditation and yoga. I met women who were on a spiritual path and shared their tips and tools with me. I journaled daily to release old emotions. I call this my time of awareness.

I took a leave of absence from my part-time job during the seven months Ellie spent at the inpatient residential treatment facility. I felt the entire family would need my full attention adjusting to Ellie's time away. My employer was so gracious and supportive of my decision, which made it even easier for me to transition from working to being home full-time and putting my family first.

I was grateful to have this time at home to focus on all my

family members, including myself. For so long, I was involved in Ellie's day-to-day care and my other priorities as a wife and parent that I didn't have much time left for me. I felt like I lost who I was and what I wanted out of my future dreams. Slowly, over time, I had faded away into the challenges of motherhood and raising a child with diagnosed mental illness.

My house was quiet during the day while Lucca, my son, was at school and Mario was at work. I didn't sit in anger or resentment for my current situation. I used this time to empower and transform myself by reading, learning new ideas, and connecting with new people. I was starting to feel some peace and control over my day.

We visited Ellie as a family at the facility every weekend. This was time to have some normalcy in an abnormal environment. The first month, we visited Ellie at the cabin where she was living. There was a particular room for family visits. The walls were blue with images painted on them by the residents; it had a couch, beanbag, and no door. It was not completely private but enough to get away from the others. We sat together for a few hours as a family and talked.

Ellie called home twice a day and would only speak with me. "Why did you put me in here?" she asked, her tears clear even through the phone. "What did I do that was so bad?"

Day after day, she begged to come home.

Day after day, my heart crumbled into pieces.

As Ellie showed she was responsible and compliant, she earned time away from the facility with her family on the weekends. We could take her out of the facility for most of the day, going to the local mall, a movie, lunch, the library, the park, or anything to feel like an average family. My heart was heavy every time we brought her back to the facility. Walking up the stairs was gut-wrenching, knowing that it meant goodbye until the following weekend. Each time, I hoped against hope that she was strong enough to continue working on her plan. This ending to the day usually included some tears and hugging.

She had visits from other family members, too—aunts, uncles, grandmas—but my dad couldn't do it. He couldn't see his grand-daughter in that environment. Ellie's papa loved her so much that it hurt his heart to see her there, and he didn't want to cry in front of her. Ellie understood and was never upset that he didn't come. I knew we were lucky to have such a supportive family.

Each week, my husband and I drove up to attend a family counseling session. The three of us sat in an office with the therapist assigned to Ellie by the facility. Ellie shared what she was learning, how she was feeling, and what she was looking forward to that week. We felt proud of how Ellie showed up in those sessions, sharing her feelings and opening up more than any other sessions we had tried in the past. We saw a different level of maturity in her. She was thriving in some ways with the structure the facility provided, under the knowledge of what was expected of her. She was also an example to the other girls in her cabin with her positive insight and support. This comes naturally for those of us who are sensitive empaths. Even when we are struggling, we give our love and support to those we see in need.

Ellie was making some changes, but we didn't feel like she was making huge strides that would change her life's direction when she returned home. She was doing the work needed to get herself out as soon as possible. This was worrisome because it felt like a last resort for her mental care, yet she was playing their game, doing what they wanted, in hopes that she could leave. I started to think about what we would do if this didn't work for her. What would be next?

As someone who enjoys research, I set out like an explorer blazing a trail to seek answers for my daughter's struggle with mental illness. We had followed the system and recommendations for years but hadn't improved her mental health. My research allowed me to learn something new, put me in control of learning, and challenged me to look outside my comfort zone. I am a seeker of truth and want to make sense of situations. So, with my own child struggling for so long, I felt the need to research childhood mental illness. I had the time and energy to devote to exploring other perspectives, and didn't have any predefined goal as to what type of information I was seeking. I was open-minded and didn't overlook information simply because it went against what I preferred to be true. I was willing to accept the truth, regardless of what information I found.

During this period of research, I also started a path of self-discovery. I had time to learn who I was on different levels and not just who I was told I was. I began to become aware of who I could be as an individual. I was opening up to a new way of looking at our family's life. We didn't have to search out experts' help from the outside for all the answers. We had what we needed within us.

Intuition is a powerful force that can guide you in making decisions. It begins as a feeling in your gut, but you can develop your awareness to recognize it wherever it shows up. Intuition is an important tool for helping you navigate life. If you listen closely, you'll become increasingly aware of what feels right.

I was not sure listening to my own inner wisdom, my intuition, would work. I questioned everything, and I second-guessed myself. But it all worked out because I decided to trust that whatever happened, it would be OK.

This feeling was so strong; it was faith. In GUS (God, Universe, and Spirit), or whatever you want to believe. I just knew we were meant to travel this journey and we would get through it no matter what.

"You can't connect the dots looking forward; you can only connect them looking backward. So, you have to trust that the dots will somehow connect in your future."—Steve Jobs

We never know where we are going but take the next step in

faith. The reason will reveal itself in the future as our experiences connect. As I look back on my journey with Ellie, I have clarity and respect for how all my dots connected. I had to learn how to listen to my intuition and move in confidence toward the unfolding path. I had to feel the intuition and give it a voice.

As I was awakening, I grew and understood my true self. I felt nudged to do something outside of the home but didn't want to return to my employer and my previous schedule, as Ellie was just a few months into her treatment. I have worked most of my adult life and always took pleasure in daily structure. I decided to join a direct sales business that would allow me to work from home and sell a product I enjoyed. I was very motivated to put my attention to something new. In little over a month, I had a large team of other direct sales consultants under me. I never saw myself as a leader. I was always the quiet one in the corner observing. I had spent my entire career supporting others. At one of the lowest points in our family's life, I felt empowered to take on a leadership role, leading others toward their goals. I felt more and more like a different person. I felt strong, energized, creative, and inspired. I embraced this sense of accomplishment that allowed my focus to veer away from my worries about Ellie.

With my new direct sales business, I worked directly with the owner and founder. I was involved in decision-making and training programs. This was different from my experience with Ellie's doctors, therapists, and psychiatrists, who gave suggestions that I followed blindly. In my new role, I was being asked what I thought about new products and ways to motivate our teams. I felt recognized for my devotion to the company.

In January 2014, one of my team members reached out to me with a message about a women's networking group.

Heather, this totally looks like something that you would be interested in, she wrote in an email. *It's a group where women support other women. —Laura*

I went to the website for more information and was immediately interested. Laura was right—it was something I would love. The group was about positive, action-forward women, with a focus on collaboration, not competition. They happened to be launching a chapter near my home in the next couple of months, so I joined right away without attending a meeting. If something feels right to me, I just do it. I felt guided toward this networking group for a reason. It was a meaningful coincidence, also known as synchronicity.

Before that chapter launched and I attended my first meeting, I was contacted by the founder of the networking group. I was totally surprised by the message she sent to me. She asked if I would be interested in applying as a managing director to open my own chapter. What?! Me? I didn't have the experience. I was a mom working for a direct sales company. Again, I jumped right in because it felt right. The founder didn't know me as a parent to Ellie, a child with mental illness; she saw me as Heather, a successful leader with a direct sales business who could lead a networking group.

I went through the application and interview process, and was offered my own chapter, which I launched in April 2014. I invited women I had never met to attend the launch of this new, amazing networking group for women. I built a leadership team of four women that I didn't know but felt connected to, and they supported me and the chapter as we grew. On the day of the launch, I spoke to a room of thirty women with the founder of the organization. *Me!* The person who would skip speech class because she was so full of anxiety and was afraid to be called on in elementary school, remember? All of this was happening while my child was away receiving treatment for mental illness.

As I launched my own chapter of this women's networking group, my husband commented, "You have your sparkle back." That was a moment of recognition that I needed. I was coming out of the darkness, and others were seeing it. I honored my intuition and inner wisdom by both joining the group and then launching a community. I would never have imagined the importance of this group when I first said yes. I was united with women who provided essential pieces to support our family's journey.

I was practicing self-love. Joining the women's networking group was a nudge toward acceptance and understanding of my true self. In leading this space, the right people came my way to give guidance. Guests and members of the group knew I was a leader with a heart, which is why they crossed my path. I didn't see it at that time, but I see now it was the plan created for me by GUS (God, Universe, and Spirit).

I received messages from my divine guidance, inner wisdom, intuition, or whatever you would like to call it. I listened and didn't question the direction in which I felt led. Sometimes we don't listen to those messages because we aren't sure how to. When you start to consciously work on your intuition, you increase your self-worth and confidence. You begin to have faith that your intuition will never let you down.

With the support of the women I met in this networking group, I started my spiritual awareness. I met with holistic practitioners, healers, speakers, coaches, authors, and businesswomen. They were sent to me for a reason; synchronicity, or divine guidance, was happening.

I started to feel comfortable enough to share pieces of my family's struggles with specific members of the group. I was given support, guidance, suggestions, and love. No judgment! The right people were in my life when I needed them. As I became more comfortable with myself and sharing more about my life with others, I was inspired to take a different path with my business and study areas I believed would be helpful to support Ellie and other families. I became a certified holistic life coach, ThetaHealer®, flower and gemstone essence practitioner, kids' nutrition specialist, and a self-love guide from The Path of Self-Love School with Christine Arylo. This is more than I would have ever dreamed for myself. It is incredible what you can accomplish with uplifting women—and a supportive husband—by your side.

I met a mom who was on a similar path, searching for a deeper understanding of her young daughter's behavior and emotions. We shared some stories about our daughters and the struggles we were experiencing. We bonded over the idea that our daughters were sensitive and gifted in a spiritual sense. She invited me to attend a drumming class at the local metaphysical center. I had no idea what "drumming" meant and had never been to a metaphysical center. This was one of my first steps toward open-mindedness. I stepped out of my comfort zone and trusted that I would enjoy this new experience.

The first time I walked in I felt uneasy and way out of my comfort zone. I met the instructor, Jayna, and the owner of the facility, Laura. They immediately made me feel comfortable. In the drumming class, I felt different; I felt open and peaceful. I would return to more and more classes at the metaphysical center and develop my spiritual gifts.

The drumming class instructor, Jayna, personally invited me to train with her in Milagros Energywork™. This is a sacred energy healing technique combining energies from the Divine, the heart, and the earth with assistance from the angelic realms. I did train with her, but it didn't feel right or in alignment after a few weeks. I told Jayna how I was feeling, and she responded, "You are a healer with words, not your hands." Look at me, now writing a book. She was right.

My commitment to understanding and accepting new ideas made all the difference in my perspective of Ellie's mental health and led me to research ideas that most others would pass by simply because they aren't conventionally accepted. I connected with people I would not usually have in my life.

Laura, the metaphysical center owner, invited me back to hold a monthly empowerment circle years later. I enjoyed my time in that space, and I felt accepted. I learned to show up as my true self and to support others in doing the same. After Ellie came home, I brought her with me to classes, and she also felt the love and support. It was fantastic to find a place where I could learn, be accepted, and teach.

After three years in a leadership role with the networking group, I listened to my intuition when I felt it was time to leave. I no longer felt in alignment with the founder and leadership of the organization. I heard with my intuition, "You are ready to move on to other things." I am thankful and blessed for all the amazing women who came into my life and the lessons I learned. One lesson learned, which was hard for me, is we outgrow things, even those that were amazing. It is essential to know when it is time to move on and not overstay.

WHEN SENSITIVE EMPATHS AREN'T AWAKE

Becoming aware and understanding that Ellie and I were sensitive empaths was life-changing. I finally understood my own daughter, a vast array of experiences and emotions started to make sense from my childhood and my parenting journey with Ellie. My daughter needed a parent who would embrace her differences and fully understand her. I needed that too.

I see that little girl sitting at the desk in elementary school, afraid to speak up for fear of being judged by others. That was me, a sensitive soul with so many feelings bombarding me at once that I felt frozen. Ellie was the little girl staring out the window in what appeared to be a daydream, who was called ADHD inattentive by doctors. As sensitive empaths we are often so busy sorting out, observing, and processing information and emotions that we lose connection with ourselves. We start to identify with everyone but ourselves. We own everyone's feelings. This can cause sensitive empaths to feel lost or overwhelmed.

I started to awaken gradually. The darkness felt like living in despair; I was trapped and sad. But the light brought feelings of peace, pleasure, and joy, and I felt like I was more of myself—my essence.

Your essence transcends the stories we tell ourselves. Living in the dark is like living in gray space without color. Living in the light feels more vibrant and alive. The best way to show your children that you love them is by learning to value yourself as a person, learning from your failures and mistakes, and healing from traumatic experiences.

INNER WORK

Inner work shines the light of awareness to your true essence or innermost being. I was so caught up in trying to be a good parent, worker, friend, partner, and so many other things, I neglected to truly see who I was. We are often taught who we are by parents, society, media, or other outside influences. When this happens, we ignore our beliefs, feelings, hopes, and desires.

As unpleasant as it may seem, unhappiness brings us to the inner work we need to do to discover our true potential. We must learn to take responsibility rather than run away or cover things up with poor behaviors. Part of the inner work I did was regarding my self-love and diving into shadow work. I had reached a point in life where I had no idea who I was, what I was doing, or why. My life seemed like a constant cycle of appointments and caring for others. I was exhausted. Then I began to look within to find the answers. Inner work allowed me to turn pain into power, dissolve shame, and turn judgment into compassion.

HIGHER VIBRATION

When Ellie returned home from her stay at the inpatient residential treatment facility, I believe she could feel a shift in me. All the transformational work I was doing for myself shifted me from a place of sadness and overwhelm to peace and love. My decisions were now being made from the heart. I used words differently to express my decisions as "I feel," instead of "I think." It was more of a feeling from my heart than a decision made from the mind. I was executing this new part of me, my intuition, and it was reflecting on Ellie. This was a critical moment in our journey because this shift allowed her a space to feel truly seen.

You have probably heard the term vibration or vibe. Our vibration is a fancy way of describing our overall state of being. Everything is energy, including you. Every cell in your body vibrates at different frequencies. Everything you think, say, and do reflects your vibrational frequency. This means your thoughts and emotions directly affect the physical world you live in. High frequency vibrations are usually associated with positive qualities and feelings like love, joy, compassion, forgiveness, or peace. Low frequency vibrations are usually associated with darker qualities and emotions like anxiety, depression, fear, anger, resentment, or hatred.

As your vibration elevates, you'll feel more in tune with yourself, your inner guidance, or your soul. You'll feel more grounded, centered, and in command of who you are. This also means when living in a lower vibrational state, you can feel disconnected from your higher self and inner guidance leading to feelings of disharmony.

Once I was on my path of spiritual awareness and awakening, my vibration elevated. With the shift of my vibration, I strengthened my intuition. I already felt very connected and in tune with my intuition, but it was even stronger. I learned to listen rather than ignore the guidance of my intuition. The shift of my vibration shifted my entire family without them really knowing what was happening.

Since families share space and communicate through both speech and nonverbal cues, this creates energy in your home. Every word you speak or facial expression you make is sending a message. When you have awareness around this idea, you can make personal shifts to elevate, and they will align with your vibration.

BOUNDARIES

A sign that you are growing in your spiritual awareness is when you start to put up boundaries. I didn't understand the importance of boundaries as I raised Ellie until later in her life, when she was around fifteen. I grew up in a household with not many rules or boundaries.

My parents were well-intentioned but had no clue about building boundaries, so they passed on their limited boundary functioning to me. My husband grew up in a home with strict boundaries and rules. So, when we came together to raise a child, we created confusion and frustration for all of us. This fueled some of Ellie's anxiety because she didn't know what to expect from her parents when it came to discipline or boundaries.

When I think of boundaries I think of a line. Sometimes it is straight and easy to draw, and other times it is jagged and difficult to explain or receive. For so long I didn't have any lines with my daughter. We were in a codependent relationship. I experienced "the good girl syndrome" to please others. I knew the pain of trying to be good and not disappoint my mother. I didn't want Ellie to experience that same feeling, so I swung the pendulum in the other direction of coddling and protecting her feelings to the point of not having boundaries. I was unaware at the time that we were sensitive empaths, and our energy and emotions were intertwined. Thanks to my awakening, I grew able to use my new self-awareness and knowledge to the benefit of my entire family, especially Ellie.

Chapter Five

THE REQUEST

I was willing to accept new ideas and research other options for the care of my daughter. This change required a willingness to commit to further actions and transform old behaviors and mindsets. I wasn't willing until I felt no other option. Pain is a great teacher and usually motivates us to change. In effect, pain creates willingness. This understanding allowed me to break old patterns and see things with fresh new perspective.

My personal desire to grow, change, and accept new experiences into my life allowed for shifts to happen within Ellie. I believe this opened the space within her to speak her truth and lean into her intuition.

Once I felt Ellie was speaking from her intuition and not her logic, I listened without shutting her down. We made changes based on what she was saying. This encouraged her to trust her intuition and build respect, after years of misleading her into therapy and treatment had broken that down in her.

A few months after returning home from her stay at the inpatient residential treatment facility, Ellie approached me while I was at my computer.

"Mom," she said, "I want to go off all my medications." I was surprised by this statement, but I looked into her eyes and knew she was serious. My stomach dropped, and I sat up in my chair, ready to dive into a conversation.

"Ellie, why do you feel this way?" I asked.

Ellie explained she was tired of feeling like a zombie. She had no feelings and felt numb. I listened and reassured her that I heard what she was saying and I was proud of her for sharing her feelings with me. I also told her I would speak with her dad and get back to her with a decision. This was a spark of her intuition. Ellie was taking the lead on this new path and requesting what she needed at age fourteen.

I had some reservations as I spoke with my husband, which came from years of using medications to care for her mental health and not knowing what she would be like off them. I felt this was a significant moment in my gut, and it deserved time and thought before it received an answer. On the other hand, I thought I knew the answer, or my intuition already knew. I spoke with my husband and shared Ellie's request. We both felt it was a scary decision but a necessary one. We decided to sit with the question for a few days instead of giving Ellie an answer right away.

In the meantime, I had a networking meeting, and one of the guests visiting was with a local bank. At the end of the meeting, she approached me and said, "I don't think I can join this group. I am a medium and the energy is too overwhelming for me." I was taken aback, as she didn't mention that she was a medium in the meeting. I felt honored that she took the time to share her feelings with me. I told her I understood and thanked her for coming.

I couldn't stop thinking about the medium from the meeting. I found the idea of a medium interesting but wasn't fully knowledgeable about what they did. I went online to search the word, and found that a medium is said to be able to bridge the physical world and the spiritual world to engage in communication with spirits. These may take the form of the deceased's spirits, spiritual beings such as angels or nature spirits, or gods.

Ellie and I have always had an interest in the paranormal. When she was young, we would watch paranormal shows on TV together. We still do! I have always been intrigued by the idea of ghosts and people with spiritual gifts.

I couldn't get the medium out of my mind. Could she provide

some answers on Ellie's mental health? Could she help us find clarity about the request Ellie had made? At this point, I thought nothing could hurt, so I made the decision to reach out to her and request a session for Ellie.

While shopping in Target with my son, I received a response about a session. The medium said she had already received a message from one of our family members that had passed. As I stood in Target, goosebumps rose on my arms, and tears welled up in the inner corner of my eyes. This felt like a sign, a confirmation affirming my decision to reach out to the medium. I scheduled a session for Ellie and me to see her in person.

On the day of our scheduled session, Lucca was in school and it was like any typical day except for the sixty minutes when Ellie and I would be sitting across from a medium. I felt excited and nervous, hoping for some answers but trying not to be too optimistic. It was hard for me to read how Ellie was feeling, but that was normal. I did give her some background information before we left for our session.

"I don't care," said Ellie, as usual, and shrugged her shoulders. At least I didn't have to fight to get her in the car. She did ask a few questions on the twenty-minute drive, which showed me she had some interest and wanted to know what to expect.

We pulled up to the medium's home near a beautiful lake. I was feeling some butterflies in my stomach but wanted to show a calm exterior for Ellie. Ellie slowly walked behind me as she often did when going into a new situation. I rang the doorbell and was greeted with a kind smile and a warm welcome into her home. Amber, the medium, directed Ellie and me to a room with two chairs on one side and one chair on the other. I let Ellie pick her chair, and then I sat in the other one next to her. Directly across from us was the medium. Ellie was quiet and I spoke up for both of us. Again, this was a typical pattern. Amber explained that she was a psychic medium, which meant she could receive messages from those that had passed and tune in to a spirit guide, angel, or a higher power.

She said a prayer before beginning, and spoke to us with her eyes closed. She asked if we had any specific questions. I told her we didn't, we just wanted whatever needed to come through to be shared. Amber knew nothing about Ellie or me, except for my business and networking group.

I don't remember everything from that session, but the most critical piece was when she said to us, "Archangel Michael is stepping forward." She then asked, "Is Ellie on any medication?"

"Yes," I responded.

"He says this child should not be on any medication. She is a bright light, with many gifts."

She continued with her reading, but that message was the most important takeaway from our session. When she was done, I told her parts of what Ellie had experienced in her life. The medium didn't remember what she had told us because she was only a conduit for the messages we received. This was a very emotional moment for me. I don't think Ellie was fully aware of how this moment was going to change her life.

The message we received from Archangel Michael through the medium was a nudge toward agreeing to Ellie's question of going off medication. This was the confirmation I needed to move confidently toward a new direction with Ellie's mental well-being.

I never told my husband about the experience Ellie and I had with the medium. I felt he wouldn't believe what we were told or would judge it. I wanted to honor it and keep it sacred. I haven't shared this story with many people because it was a message for Ellie and me. Sharing this with you is important so you can understand how our journey unfolded and how that one message played a huge part in our decision to go another direction.

The medium's reading with Ellie opened my eyes and changed my perception of the spirit world. This was real life, not an experience on a TV show or movie. I felt as if I had some power in the decision-making for my child. For so long, I felt the need to follow the guidance of other recommendations for my child's care. This was going to be different.

I was feeling confident in myself as I grew on a personal level. I think my husband could also feel this strength and determination, which allowed him to feel comfortable with the new direction we took with Ellie's care. He was never entirely on board with the prescriptions from the start, and supported what I felt would be a good decision.

Please seek medical guidance if you choose to go off any prescribed medication. This was our family's personal decision. I don't make medical recommendations.

Our first step was to wean Ellie off her prescription medications. We decided to do this with the information provided by our doctor. We slowly implemented a gradual decrease in doses over weeks. I was still on a leave of absence from my job, and it was summer, so Ellie was not in school. This allowed me to monitor her side effects and, if needed, take her to the doctor. It took about a month to give her body time to adjust. Ellie experienced minimal side effects like stomachaches, nausea, headaches, insomnia, and anxiety. These were the same experiences she had in her daily life anyway with her prescriptions, so Ellie didn't notice much of a difference. As the months went on and the medicines were out of her system, I noticed the brightness in her eyes return. They no longer looked dark to me like they had when she was on medication. My Ellie was returning! The Ellie who enjoyed life, her friends, and family. I knew we made the right decision for our child.

Ellie was still adjusting to her life at home after six months in treatment. She was involved with the family and seemed to have matured while at the facility. Part of this newfound behavior could have been due to the skills she learned and the motivation not to return to another facility, as well as the lack of prescription medications in her system.

As Ellie came off her medications, which kept her in a state of low vibrations, she began the process of her own awakening. She started to see dark masses, shadows, and hear voices. Some nights, the voices were highly active, and others, there was nothing. Ellie saw mists, masts, and shapes of beings, as well as shimmering objects that appeared like glittery particles. Once, we returned home as a family from an event, and Ellie walked into the house first.

"Mom, did you see that?"

I didn't see anything out of the ordinary. Ellie pulled me aside and told me she saw an outline of a person. It was a spirit, and she felt it was not harmful. It was gone quickly. I told her I was thankful to her for sharing that with me. I wanted to be a safe space for Ellie to share and not feel judged. I listened without reaction or advice, just held space for her to be heard. Then we moved along with our day.

Some experiences were frightening for her. I remember one night she came running into our room, as we all slept, to say, "Mom, I saw something scary. It was black, and it was by my bed." I comforted her and told her it would be OK. She and I walked down the stairs to her bedroom with me in the lead. Ellie's hand held tightly to the back of my shirt. I approached her room, not in fear, but with a strong sense of power and strength. I would not allow anything to harm my child. I told Ellie anything bad or dark would dissipate if we called on God and the angels. Darkness fears the light. Together, standing in the middle of her room, that is just what we did, and we also said a prayer. I asked Ellie how she felt, and she said, "I think it is gone, it feels OK now." She agreed to sleep in her room for the rest of the night, knowing I was only a few stairs away if she needed to call me.

The following day, I thought of a contact I had made. Jessica was a Master Healer, and I felt what happened to Ellie was spiritual, not a mental illness. It was the weekend, but I messaged Jessica and shared our experience from that night. I asked her for guidance supporting Ellie.

She messaged back: *I could see her today if you are willing to bring her to my office.*

I was, but I needed Ellie's consent. The spiritual world was all so new to her, and I was not sure how Ellie would feel. Ellie agreed, and we went to Jessica's office that afternoon. Jessica explained that Ellie had had an attachment to her since the age of two. The release of the attachment was overwhelming, and observing Jessica as she waved her hands and spoke loudly over my daughter was an intense experience for both me and Ellie. We didn't visit Jessica again. It is important to find a healer that feels right to you.

We are still learning, and Ellie continues to have some experiences, though not to the extent she did at the beginning of her awakening. She might be blocking her gifts. If so, they will come knocking at her door again. If so, I will be there to support her. It takes a parent shifting and becoming an awakened parent to honor the journey with their child.

Taking Ellie off her prescription medication was the best solution for her. This was done carefully and tailored to our child's needs. This is an individual or family decision and should not be taken lightly. Do your research, listen inwardly, listen to your child, and find the best direction for your family. One of my goals with this book is to bring awareness to other options. There is no universal solution to mental illness. Just as prescriptions should not be the only option, our situation should not be the only answer to every mental health situation.

"Some changes look negative on the surface, but you will soon realize that space is being created in your life for something new to emerge."
—*Eckhart Tolle*

This was also the time we started introducing Ellie to holistic modalities, which helped relieve her minimal medication withdrawal symptoms like headaches and sleep issues, and introduced us to a new way of living. We used meditation, essential oils, and flower essences.

I was introduced to flower essences by a woman who attended one of my monthly networking meetings. She was sharing about her business, a shop offering high-quality crystals, stones, handcrafted energetic mists, and more. She spoke about the use of crystals and stones as a tool for anxiety and emotional healing. I felt grateful, like she was speaking to me in that moment.

A few weeks later, I went to her store, intending to purchase a few crystals for Ellie. I thought it would be fun and couldn't hurt in any way, so why not give it a try. While there, I was able to share more about Ellie and her past experiences. I didn't mind sharing parts of our story because I searched for any kind of guidance or resource. I talked about how Ellie didn't like to leave our house and how she took on the emotions of others. This is when I first learned the word "empath." An empath, I learned that day, can sense the emotions of others around them because they are so attuned. This experience can leave them confused by which emotion is theirs or someone else's. I was so surprised that someone understood my daughter on a different level. I purchased crystals along with flower essences to help Ellie with the symptoms of being an empath. Ellie wasn't sure what a crystal or some flower essences in a bottle would do to help her, but she took them in stride and was willing to try. Ellie started to call the flower essences her "positive potion" as it allowed her to feel a shift. She started asking to go shopping with me and attended family meals at restaurants. This was so amazing, as she hadn't wanted to leave the house in such a long time.

The change in Ellie was so great that it affirmed our decision to adopt a different lifestyle. We are now living a life of mainly holistic modalities. She does see a medical doctor for her annual exam and as needed for medical issues. She does still experience anxiety and depression at times, which I think is partly from being an empath and partly from when she neglects to practice self-care or use her coping skills.

In 2018, Ellie experienced pain in her chest, clamminess, and nausea while driving to pick up my son from school. She said, "Mom, bring me to the hospital." I was unable to because I had to pick up my son, so I called for an ambulance to meet us at the school. We still believe in the importance of the medical system to care for us. The EMTs were so kind and provided tests, but nothing was physically wrong. It was a panic attack. As sensitive empaths, we can feel so profoundly that we can get to an overwhelmed state, leading to panic. We still need to seek out care from mainstream medicine.

Ellie no longer wanted to see anyone for therapy as she felt it didn't help, and she was tired of telling the same stories repeatedly. She began to work with healers and coaches to heal past trauma and look toward the future. All her experiences made her a strong person, and she began to firmly believe in the support of family. This also led her to understand that there is another way to look at mental illness. Ellie no longer hides her struggles but owns them as part of her. This is a journey that will continue her whole life.

Years later, I brought up the time we visited the medium and the decision to go off her prescription medication. Ellie didn't remember asking to stop her medication. This was when I knew the message came through her by spiritual guidance. She spoke it to me but wasn't aware that she did. If she wouldn't have been open to allowing this message or receiving it, I don't know where we would be right now.

Ellie asking to go off her prescription medications was one of my *aha* moments. That moment caused a significant shift in my perspective of the care for her mental health. The change in perspective allowed me to see her mental illness in a different light. It moved me to seek other means of support and holistic options and find hope for her future.

Someone once said, "The definition of insanity is doing the same thing over and over again but expecting different results."

This is a common thread for most people during their life. Something must shake you awake before you can make a change. The reason for this shake-up is to give you a wake-up call. Wake-up calls cause us to question everything, from the meaning of our lives and relationships to how we spend our time. For me, it caused me to question the care of my child. A wake-up call can feel like something is shattering. Some of us need several wake-up calls before we respond. Once you allow for the space to receive the wake-up call, you can take the step forward. Healing is a lifelong process. There are no shortcuts. It requires digging deep into your soul, exploring the unknown parts of your emotional heart, and showing up for yourself when you're in pain. Allowing yourself time to really heal is the only way to find true transformation. It requires you to allow space for possibilities to emerge, have faith with the unknown, listen to your intuition, be willing to dig deep into the problem, and commit to seeing it through.

We step out of our comfort zone so we can grow deeper. Sometimes we go through a cold winter so that our roots will go down deep to our source. Other times, we enjoy a spring season of abundant rain. No matter what season we are in, GUS (God, Universe, and Spirit) is there with us. Do not miss the purpose of the process. GUS does not shake you to torment you, but to awaken you.

It can be scary and challenging to try different approaches to the problems in our lives, even when we are unhappy. The stories that we tell ourselves about our lives become a fundamental aspect of our identities. That might also be why it's so hard to make changes. These stories are comfortable, and they include our very thoughts, emotions, and behaviors. For me, I was the parent of a child with mental illness. We kept down the same path for seven years, and it never got smoother, only bumpier and more troubling. The cycle continued until I chose to work on myself. I started to listen to my own intuition and that of my child. I explored my own spiritual path. I surrounded myself with a community that was supportive of mind-body-spirit and personal development. I healed old wounds and practiced self-love, allowing Ellie's space to elevate and open to her needs. Ellie spoke up. Her words shook me awake, and I started to think differently. If you want different results, you must try different approaches.

When you change your perspective and look at the world through a different lens, it can be uncomfortable. We are walking an unknown path and we must trust in our faith. When you follow your intuition, you are not only demonstrating faith in yourself but also in GUS. We must overcome our doubts and fears, no matter how difficult this may seem. I am an example of this truth and how it has transformed my family's life. You can do this as well.

Part Two

PUTTING TOGETHER THE PIECES

Guidance and Lessons

Chapter Six

ANOTHER WAY

Ellie asking to go off her prescription medications was one of my *aha* moments, which caused a significant shift in my perspective of her mental health care. If not for that moment, I am not sure where we would be today, and I would not have these messages to share with you. It allowed me to see her mental illness in a different light. It moved me to seek other means of support and holistic options, and find hope for her future.

We have learned many lessons that we have taken forward with us. Some I have already shared with you. I hold these lessons to be sacred and honor the journey that brought about our transformation.

It all starts with us not hiding our experiences. We need to be comfortable sharing our feelings and thoughts because the secret to happiness is through acceptance. We need to come together to end the stigma of mental health because secrets destroy lives. In sharing our stories, we can rebuild confidence and help others recognize they're not alone.

Labels, treatments, and medications are meant to lessen symptoms and make those around them happy. I am not one to support the labeling of children, but I understand labels serve a purpose when communicating for the proper treatment, assessment, or testing. Depending on your insurance and school policy, you may need a diagnosis before therapy or other services begin.

It is important to realize that labels are just labels, not the sum of who the child is. When my daughter describes herself as crazy,

I don't let that label become the sum of all she is. She is a girl with a lot of strengths and unique characteristics.

DOCTOR CARE

We are not one-dimensional beings, so our approach to mental health shouldn't be either. We should look at what works best for our family. This could mean looking at multidimensional or multi-disciplinary approaches among psychology, psychiatry, Western medicine, alternative medicine, and holistic modalities in combination with what is needed for your child. Some may not even need a psychiatric intervention at all. Consider options before you medicate your child. I didn't know of all the amazing opportunities and research about other causes for what appears as mental illness. The holistic approach considers the whole person—mind, body, and spirit, just as we did later with Ellie!

Symptoms of mental illnesses could be caused by various issues that aren't shared with you when visiting your pediatrician. When searching for reasons behind your child's behavior, research other possibilities such as nutrition, stress, thyroid, sleep, allergies, vitamin deficiency, highly sensitive child, or empathic gifts. Often the first diagnosis received for kids is generalized anxiety disorder (GAD) or ADHD. These diagnoses are given after a fifteen-minute appointment where symptoms are described and the health professional concludes from a checklist. Often parents walk away with prescription medication. There are no brain scans, blood tests, or anything definite used during diagnosis. Because they don't know better, many parents settle for this diagnosis before considering an alternative or underlying issue, just like I did with Ellie in the beginning.

I understand why parents choose medication. It is a Band-Aid, and it feels better than watching their child hurting. I know I went in that direction. Please realize the medication is helping manage the anxiety, but it is not healing it. Recognizing how and why a symptom started is necessary for healing. If you understand anxiety, you can prevent it or reduce its impact and begin the healing process.

Do you wonder why more and more children are receiving a diagnosis of ADHD, ADD, anxiety, depression, suicidal ideation, bipolar disorder, or other mental illnesses? We are in crisis!

We aren't seeing our children's symptoms from any other perspective. We aren't provided with optimal solutions when we visit the doctor's office.

I believe in using our medical system and holistic health care together. Holistic health care focuses on the patient's wellness and prevention of illness rather than treating the symptoms. The medical system diagnoses and treats patients. Bringing these two together is the best solution for the patient. There is no one-size-fits-all treatment plan.

I believe in balance when talking with doctors. I don't follow their advice blindly, but instead weigh it against my intuition. I speak my truth and advocate for myself. It's important to be an active participant in your life, rather than just a passive spectator. Being an active participant requires that you put yourself first and that you trust yourself. Also, act with intention, even when it goes against what everyone else is doing.

SCHOOL SYSTEM

In seventh grade, Ellie struggled with grades. We had conversations with her teachers about creating an IEP (individual education plan) or putting her in a special program with other kids who didn't fit into the norm. Our school system is not built for these special kids. These options didn't feel suitable for our child. I think these conversations made Ellie feel even worse, because it was a confirmation of her feeling different. Kids who are a distraction or don't fit into the typical classroom environment are put into another space because we don't know how to help them. Our school system has hardly changed over the past two hundred years. This is an aged, broken, and declining structure.

Our school system is built on the idea that everybody's brain works similarly, and the job of the students is to retain information. We are all unique, but our current schools fail to take that into account. The system is over-prescriptive and risks stigmatizing any child who doesn't fit into one of the predefined categories. When students have a unique talent, they should be embraced.

I think our educational system fails some of our children and doesn't do enough to nurture creativity. Seemingly, hating school is commonplace among sensitive and gifted kids. This just shows how deeply our educational system is inadequate, and how damaging it is to children. We must acknowledge our inadequacies in our current educational system if we are to improve the lives of our children. It's time to acknowledge the problems, discuss solutions, and move forward so everyone benefits.

We should not blame teachers for our failing education system. Most teachers care deeply about their students and are frustrated by the challenges they face every day. Our education system is flawed; we need to work together as teachers, students, parents, and administrators to make education better.

Education is important in today's world, but it doesn't necessarily have to be traditional. Each of us is different and each of us needs different skills and knowledge to develop to our full potential. If we have a talent, we should be allowed to nurture it. While we are in school, our uniqueness is simply collapsing under the school curriculum.

My daughter went to an online school that encouraged her to develop her own strengths and talents. We need to wake up to this idea. We need a collaborative approach to teaching that is sensitive to the needs of each student.

An educational system that creates an environment in which students are allowed to think independently, develop their own talents, and not be afraid to make mistakes, while encouraging individuality and creativity, would be so much better than the current model. The private high school my son is attending is making strides toward creating a space for all students to feel safe and heard. I'm not sure if this is also happening in the public-school environment. I hope so!

Highly gifted children are frequently mislabeled with ADHD, autism, depression, or bipolar disorder. Yet sometimes, being gifted effectively hides these same conditions. Gifted children often feel and experience the world far more intensely. They can experience rapid mood swings, sensitivity, apprehension, feelings of inadequacy, and over empathizing with others. Gifted children often display ADHD-like symptoms because they are bored with what other kids their age are doing. Gifted behaviors can be seen as insufficient attention, boredom, daydreaming, and low tolerance for tasks that seem irrelevant.

Many spiritually gifted or empathic children are brilliant, but it is the constant distraction that causes them problems. They sense everything, so even the blinking of a light or the noise of a dog barking down the block can throw them off.

It is important that educators and parents of students who face challenges or are gifted alike seek to identify the unique ways of learning for everyone. It is important to advocate for their educational needs. They might not thrive in the cookie cutter curriculum to meet their diverse needs. Education should be an engaging and meaningful experience for all students.

ELLIE'S FUTURE

Ellie attended an online high school from ninth to twelfth grade. This decision was hard for her dad and me. Ellie advocated for herself as she didn't want to return to a public school. She wanted to be fully online and receive an education in a space she felt comfortable. We wanted her to experience "normal" high school life, but we were reminded that our daughter had already overcome so much, and we didn't want to put her back in a space that would create stress.

Ellie graduated from her online high school in June 2018. This was an emotional day, as it is for all parents, but I wasn't sure I would ever see her standing in cap and gown. In the depths of her mental illness struggles, her future was grim. Would she end up homeless, in a facility, or even dead? When you have lived through a dark journey with your child you learn to celebrate everyday life and not take anything for granted.

A few months after Ellie's graduation, our family moved from the home where we had lived for eighteen years. My husband had lived in that house his whole life, and it was finally time to move on to something new. We found a house that was meant for us, and all adjusted perfectly to our new home.

A few months after moving in, Ellie complained of being lightheaded. She had frequent chest pains and difficulty breathing. This would occur randomly, and I didn't notice a pattern. I thought it must be something to do with her heart, so I scheduled an appointment with her doctor. The doctor requested an EKG and blood work, and Ellie returned to the doctor to get the results.

The doctor, whom we had never seen before and didn't know Ellie's background, said, "You have panic disorder. We can give you a prescription medication and see how that helps you."

I saw tears filling Ellie's eyes. Here we go again! But this time, we were armed with knowledge. We had choices, and didn't have to follow the doctor's suggestions. I told the doctor we would discuss it and get back to her. Ellie and I had a conversation, and she decided that medication was not what she wanted. By now, she had a full toolbox of coping skills, and this was a reminder she needed to use these tools and skills as an empath. The changes she was experiencing were bringing up new feelings and some fear. For Ellie, knowing panic disorder was the cause of her feelings empowered her to use her tools.

What the future holds for my daughter is different than I imagined. At this moment, she is twenty-one and living at home, not knowing what she will do next. It is hard to balance between wanting to push her toward something—education, or a job—and accepting that it's OK for her to be where she is.

Sensitive or empathic children grow up to be sensitive or empathic adults. This is not something they outgrow. They become more mature and have awareness around their needs if they have parents supporting them and giving guidance. Sensitivity is not weakness, but the power to see and feel things intensely. Our sensitive kids need understanding, love, and support. They don't need to be fixed, as I learned from my own child. What they do need is to be accepted and understood for the fantastic people they are.

I see a shift happening. More and more people are opening, accepting, and learning about all the gifts their special children have to offer. The more we as a community of parents speak out loud, the more the truth will be heard, and society will adjust. Open yourself to your child's gifts and honor them. You are your child's best advocate. Children are born with unique gifts every day. They must be nurtured, understood, and dealt with positively. As a parent of a gifted child, we might not know where to turn for support, but one thing you should know is you are not alone. The number of children displaying gifts is growing. Many gifted children are incredibly sensitive and empathic, and when they're unable to share their strong emotions with others, they're left feeling vulnerable, confused, or hurt. Therefore, we need awareness, compassion, and change.

A QUICK CONVERSATION ON PSYCHIATRIC DRUGS

Ellie was eight years old when she was prescribed her first dose of a psychiatric drug. At first, being hopeful and open to a prescription, we felt the Prozac was moderately helpful. Over time we saw her moods continue or worsen, so we searched out additional help and testing. But as we were given more diagnoses and enacted more changes in Ellie's care, it became harder for us to accept everything we were told at face value. As parents, we try to do the best for our children. In our case, we listened to our doctors' recommendations, and they did their best with their knowledge of the symptoms provided. At one point, we were told by a psychiatrist that medication is trial and error.

I don't want my child to experience the error, and I think she did along the way, even with the best of intentions.

According to Psychcentral.com, "One in ten of America's children has an emotional disturbance such as attention deficit hyperactivity disorder, depression or anxiety, that can cause unhappiness for the child and problems at home, at play, and at school. Many of these children will be taken by their parents to their family physician or pediatrician, or, in many cases, a specialist in child mental health. The child will be carefully evaluated and may begin some type of therapy. There are many treatment options available. Choosing the right treatment for your child is important. Each child is different. At times, psychotherapies, behavioral strategies, and family support may be amazingly effective. In some cases, medications are needed to help the child become more able to cope with everyday activities."

Psychiatric drugs play their role in treatment for some children. Please do your own research and decide if this is the route best for you or your child. I feel our brightest kids—our sensitive kids, who are not of the "normal"—are being numbed by psychiatric drugs, causing them to feel like zombies.

Our current mental health care system isn't progressive enough to tolerate the evolution of our sensitive children. It appears that the first line of treatment is medication, when in fact it should be the last resource after considering other options.

The FDA has required several antidepressant drugs to now carry a "black-box" warning, alerting doctors and consumers that the medications may increase suicidal behavior in children with depression, and that the risk of using antidepressants must be carefully balanced with the need.

From the ages of twelve to fourteen, my daughter was taking two prescriptions at the same time that had "black-box" warnings. My husband and I were not informed of the severity of her medications by the prescribing doctor. I also didn't fully educate myself on the side effects, as I relied on her doctors' guidance. I am surprised she survived given the "black-box" warning and the behaviors she exhibited.

When Ellie was in seventh grade and seeing a new therapist in the school, she switched to Cymbalta for her prescription medication. Therapists can't prescribe medication, so we were referred to a psychiatrist from her clinic. I did agree to this change, but looking back, I didn't have all the facts about how unsafe this was for my child.

So, was it a coincidence that Ellie experienced suicidal ideation and depression after the switch in medication? I believe it was not. She was not getting better on her other prescription, but she wasn't worse either. This switch was made due to the length of time she was on her current medication (five years), the knowledge that her behavior was not changing, and that we were seeing a new therapist. But her new prescription started a darker turn of events, leading to the climax of our journey.

I understand that some people do need prescription medication to treat mental illness, but we were close to losing our child, either to the mental health system or death. I feel it is best for everyone to do their own research and ask questions before making any decisions.

Chapter Seven

UNDERSTANDING THE HIGHLY SENSITIVE AND EMPATHIC CHILD

I was often called too sensitive as a child, which caused me to avoid certain situations or groups, observe more than speak up, blend in with others, and feel lonely even when showing a happy face.

I could sense those same intense feelings in Ellie even when she was a young child. I didn't realize that being sensitive was a gift. It wasn't something to suppress but something to nurture into greatness. I didn't accept who Ellie was as a child and who she could become. I tried to model her into someone else, and that caused disconnection and a lack of trust between us. Ellie and I can bounce our energy and emotions off each other. If I am stressed or anxious, she will say to me, "Mom, calm down, I can feel that you are stressed." She brings awareness to me, so I can then use tools to calm myself, which in turn reduces what she is feeling. This is an example of an empathic person's daily experience. Imagine you are an eight-year-old child in a classroom with twenty or thirty other children, plus a teacher, all with different personalities and feelings. This sounds like anxiety or overwhelm.

As an empath, Ellie could sense stomachaches, aggression, sadness, headaches, and all the emotions that everyone around her was feeling. As I look back, I can see why Ellie was avoiding school even though she had friends and liked learning. She didn't know how to explain what she was experiencing at school. I sympathized with her aggression when she returned home after school, or when she had stomachaches and migraines. Our home was a safe space to release all the energy she carried from the day.

How do you distinguish between a highly sensitive child and an empath? And what is the importance of knowing the difference? According to Dr. Elaine Aron, one of the pioneers in studying sensitivity, "The highly sensitive person/child (HSP/HSC) has a sensitive nervous system. They are more aware of subtleties in his/her surroundings and are more easily overwhelmed when in a highly stimulating environment."

Empaths take the experience of the highly sensitive child to another level. Unlike highly sensitive children, empaths can sense subtle energy and absorb it from other people. Some empaths also have profound spiritual and intuitive experiences which is not commonly associated with being a highly sensitive child.

Being a highly sensitive child and an empath are not mutually exclusive; you can be both. Many highly sensitive children are also empaths. To put it simply, highly sensitive people pick up sensory stimuli, and empaths also pick up on energy.

THE CHARACTERISTICS OF A HIGHLY SENSITIVE CHILD (HSC) OR HIGHLY SENSITIVE PERSON (HSP)

Not all highly sensitive children are the same, but your child may . . .

- Feel things deeply and can be easily overstimulated in their environment.

- Often become overwhelmed by sensory overload. These children dislike loud noises, may be sensitive to tags or zippers in clothing, and may dislike more scents than other children.[4]

- Be gifted in many ways: compassion, empathy, creativity, and usually above the normal range intellectually.

- Pick up on subtleties in gesture and tone as well as the words coming out of other people's mouths.[5]

- Feel highly emotional. All kids can be emotional but a highly sensitive child may cry when they are hungry, sad, upset, excited, or happy. They may cry during sad parts in movies or get scared easier. A stern look from you could reduce them to tears.

- Dislike change. While many kids don't like change, a highly sensitive child will often shut down when forced to change routine. They may get anxious, angry, depressed, or even scared.

- Be hard on themselves, holding themselves to a very high standard. They may beat themselves up about getting something wrong.

- Worry or wonder about things that aren't deemed age-appropriate, such as death, or what will happen when they become adults. They are more sensitive to weather conditions and natural disasters.

- Prefer to play alone. They enjoy quiet, peaceful play.

- Pick up on things other children their age don't. They can also be very curious and constantly looking for answers.

- Need frequent breaks from the routine busyness of life, especially after a particularly social day.

- Love animals. HSCs often develop a special bond with animals, or are very sensitive to their needs.[6]

- Have a keen sense of observation and know how to read people well. They observe character traits and gather an accurate story of who the person is.

- Take things personally. For your child, being highly emotional means everything that happens is personal.

- Be well-behaved. Sensitive kids are well-behaved and also expect to be in similar surroundings. They don't understand when other children misbehave or aren't nice to them.

THE EMPATHIC CHILD

"An Empath refers to someone who takes empathy a significant step further. An empath can literally feel and take on other people's feelings as if they are experiencing those feelings themselves." —Dr. Judith Orloff

An empathic child is a child who is good at reading others' emotions and adjusting their behavior accordingly. In contrast, a highly sensitive child is a child who feels easily overwhelmed by this process. Have you considered the possibility that your child may be an empath or spiritually gifted? The traits of spiritually gifted and empathic children usually include being sensitive, intelligent, distracted, intuitive, and wise.

Do they seem to take on the energy of the room? Do they seem easily upset by things that do not upset other kids? Do they reach out to those in need? If any of this seems true for your child, you might have an empathic child with a spiritual gift.

I have realized that I am a sensitive empath raising a sensitive empath, gifted child. Sensitive and empathic children have a sharpened awareness of people and situations around them. Because empathic people absorb so much stimulation from the environment, they are more susceptible to feelings of anxiety. If you're an empath, you can probably intuit whether your child is, too.

In addition to the traits of the highly sensitive child, the empathic child may show some or all of these characteristics:

• Feels others' emotions as if these emotions were their own.

• Quiet, shy, introverted, withdrawn.

• May be perceived as a slow learner only because the child needs to understand the depth of something first.[7]

• Seems to read your mind. Knows what you want before you ask.

The Empathic Spectrum below was taken from *The Empath's Survival Guide* by Judith Orloff, MD.

According to Dr. Orloff, "If you think about this distinction in terms of an empathic spectrum, empaths are on the highest end, highly sensitive people are a little lower on the spectrum, and people with strong empathy but who are not HSPs or empaths are

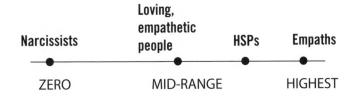

in the middle. Narcissists, sociopaths, and psychopaths, who often suffer from 'empathy deficit disorders,' are at the lowest end of the spectrum."[8]

ARE HIGHLY SENSITIVE KIDS PSYCHIC?

At this point in Ellie's life, she doesn't want to be considered a psychic, medium, or intuitive. That might change as she furthers her own understanding of her gifts. It is helpful as a parent to understand and support our children in these gifts. Our empathic children probably won't be happy in a career as an accountant or business manager. They will probably find comfort in something like working with animals or helping others. Being an empath is a gift as a healer, especially because empaths have strong intuitive skills and love to give to others. A healer is someone that desires to be of service in the world. It can be healing others with their hands, words, music, art, or their gift to share with others from a space of love.

Some empaths have spiritual and intuitive experiences. I want to clarify some of these words because they can be confusing.

According to Rebecca Rosen, "Psychics tune into people's energy or objects by feeling or sensing elements of their past, present, and future. Simply put, psychics rely on their basic sense of intuition and psychic ability to gather information for the person being read."[9]

Intuition is an unexpected feeling or sense about a situation or person. We all have intuition, but intuitive people are particularly adept at deciphering information that comes from the unconscious mind. They pay attention to these insights or feelings, and in doing so are becoming increasingly refined in this communication channel.

I used the term medium in an earlier story. According to Rosen, "A medium uses his or her psychic or intuitive abilities to see past, present, and future events by tuning into the spirit energy surrounding a person. This means mediums rely on nonphysical energy outside of themselves for the information relevant to the person being read."[10]

If you notice your child having psychic or spiritual experiences, don't dismiss them. Talk to them about it and ask questions. Learn about the metaphysical world and let your child know they can always talk to you. These are opportunities for a conversation and growth.

Let's avoid limiting our children with conventional thinking. After all, they are sacred beings, and we are their parents. If you're open and understanding, you'll notice your children's gifts early on, giving you a chance to provide a loving, supportive space for them to grow. It is empowering for both you and your child to know if they are a highly sensitive child or empath so you can parent them the way they need, understand them fully, and guide them toward being a well-adjusted adult.

> *"It is primarily parenting that decides whether the expression of sensitivity will be an advantage or a source of anxiety."* —Elaine Aron, PhD

PARENTING THE HIGHLY SENSITIVE CHILD AND EMPATH

According to Psychology Today, "Parenting a highly sensitive child"—and empath—"can be extremely rewarding, challenging, and exhausting. Sometimes all at once!" But there are a few ways you can make the journey easier on all of you:

- See sensitivity as a gift. It's easy to get frustrated and angry with your child if they continually cry, withdraw, and shy away from typical social situations. Instead of viewing your "sensitive" child as flawed, see them as having a special gift.

Sensitivity is typical of creative artists, innovators, and children who are talented in various ways.

- Don't use harsh discipline. Speak calmly even when upset. Ask your child to do something instead of yelling at them to do it. Harsh punishment can cause emotional melt-downs and outbursts.

- Focus on your child's strengths, and remember that your highly sensitive child is an incredibly talented being. Train yourself to see your child's strengths first—such as creativity, perceptiveness, and kindness—and it will be easier for you to accept their challenges.

- Understanding. Embracing your child as a highly sensitive child is the most important thing you can do for them. Many parents, like me, want to change them into less sensitive, normal kids. Instead, accept your child's sensitivity as part of your shared journey—whether you are highly sensitive or not.

- Be open and honest with them. They will know and sense if you are lying to them. This doesn't mean sharing all of your problems with them, but rather acknowledging your struggles in an age-appropriate way. Take time to explain things to your child, and reassure them you have things under control so they don't need to worry.

- Allow for quiet time. Your child needs space to unwind. Give them time to relax. Let them have some quiet time in their room to engage in an activity they enjoy.

- Create a routine. A consistent routine and predictable

structure are something a highly sensitive child needs to be happy. Most HSCs do not like to be surprised, so routines benefit them. Often HSCs have anxiety about the unknown or change, so knowing what to expect will help them feel more in control.

• Creative outlet. Highly sensitive kids are typically very creative and have great imaginations. Encouraging creativity and providing them opportunities to create will help them express themselves, work toward a goal, and build confidence.[11]

Children around three to five years old often demonstrate an ability to see and hear things that adults cannot sense. If you find this hard to imagine, ask yourself this: How many children have you known that had imaginary friends?

When my daughter reached eight years old, we saw a shift in her behavior. This shift is typical for highly sensitive and empathic children; as they approach seven or eight, they start to mature emotionally and begin to understand fairness. As a parent, offer encouragement and support through acceptance. I am a parent who didn't accept or understand her child. I did the opposite, and pushed Ellie toward being someone else. This caused a variety of issues that thrust us into a long journey to healing and understanding.

Around their teenage years, expectations can be a heavy burden for our HSCs. These years are a critical time for an HSC, as they will decide if their life will be ruled by fear or love. If a child or teen sees or hears in the spirit realm, they may act out because they feel overwhelmed and don't know how to express what they are experiencing. If the child's concerns are repeatedly dismissed, they may feel isolated and fearful.

No wonder so many youths are numbing themselves with drugs

and alcohol, or ending their lives because it is too much for them to handle. I can't stand by and watch this happen. Many of these children, youths, and young adults are sensitive. They have been either misdiagnosed or misunderstood. It is time to start supporting our children and following our intuition and the intuition of our children.

It can be exhausting to be an empath, especially for adults. When you think about how it feels to experience the energy of others without having the words to explain what you're experiencing as a child, it makes sense that this could cause anxiety, depression, behavior issues, or unexplainable illness.

Our children are sensitive, intuitive, and empathic, which causes challenges and could be seen or diagnosed as a mental illness. I feel some are misdiagnosed by professionals who don't have the knowledge about highly sensitive children, empaths, or spiritually gifted children. These symptoms are mistaken to be signs of mental health issues.

Chapter Eight

BECOMING AN ADVOCATE

I kept my voice silent as I followed all the doctors, therapists, psychologists, and psychiatrists who made suggestions for my daughter's care. After Ellie's return from the residential treatment facility, I realized through my own healing journey that I had a voice and needed to speak up for my child's care. More than that, my child had a voice that needed to be heard.

It was time to advocate for my child. It was time to question those I saw in authority and seek a different healing path for her. I could no longer sit quietly and see Ellie struggle. I overcame shyness and gained the self-confidence to advocate for my child. Now, I am ready to support other children and their families.

Advocating is speaking or acting on behalf of yourself or another to improve the quality of life. This includes needs, thoughts, feelings, safety, and rights as a human being.

I was not confident in myself or my parenting. I never thought about *what*, exactly, my role was as a parent. My spouse and I never had conversations about how we would parent or our goals with our children. We were making it up along the way, being reactive instead of proactive. Parenting is a never-ending job that has its own demands, rewards, and challenges.

I was not always a great advocate for my child. As a first-time parent, I found myself going along with the "professionals," blindly following them because they were the experts. This was partially why I did not ask too many questions when I received a treatment plan for Ellie's care. I didn't like conflict and found confronting authority difficult. It was easier for me to accept and apply. So I stayed quiet.

I thought being quiet was protecting myself from uncomfortable situations. When I was in fifth grade, I had a horrible earache the night of a dance recital. I told my mom I didn't think I could go to the recital because my ear hurt so badly.

In an angry tone, she said to me, "Your dad and I will go anyway." I felt I was being punished for having an earache. They did go, and I stayed home alone in excruciating pain, yelling out and rolling on the floor. The following day, I found bloody drainage on my pillow. My eardrum had ruptured. This was a common theme for me growing up. I learned to handle most situations independently or ask my dad for support.

I never thought of myself as an advocate until I started writing this book. I was a mom doing what I felt was best for my child. Advocating is not a one-time thing or moment in life, it is an ever-expanding practice. In my writing, I am using words to advocate for sensitive, empathic, and intuitive children. I see how being an advocate for Ellie was an essential step to helping her achieve health.

You know your child better than anyone else, so speak up and continue until you feel you have what you need to support your child. When you're dealing with teachers or doctors, remember that they're working from a generalized perspective while you know your child's particular nuances. You must be an advocate for your child since you know what's best for them. As an advocate for your child, become an expert in your child's needs. The best way to achieve this is to study your child's mental, emotional, spiritual, and physical needs. As parents, we can learn to grow and heal with our children.

If you have concerns, meet with a professional for their opinion, listen, ask questions, and—I can't emphasize this enough—ask more questions. Most importantly, listen to your intuition along with what you were given from the professionals. Our inner wisdom and intuition as parents are more often than not correct.

During the seven years that Ellie struggled with mental illness, I listened to all the other outside voices telling me how to care for my child. It came to a crucial point after Ellie had been in a partial hospitalization facility for five days. On the day of her release, the facility recommended that she continue with their intensive outpatient program, which she had already tried and found unsuccessful. We, as a family, decided she would not continue. We had to sign a document stating we knew we were going against the doctor's recommendation. We trusted our intuition and felt we were making the best decision for her. These different treatment facilities were changing her and not for the positive. Saying no to the doctors was the first step in becoming advocates for our child.

At the inpatient residential treatment facility, Ellie had to advocate for herself. She had to speak up for herself, participate in the program, and meet all the goals set for her so she could return home. She did a fantastic job and came home a stronger person, but I know she is still carrying hurt from this experience. This was the last time we sought support from the mental health field. If we felt we needed to reach out to receive services for Ellie, we would. Now, Ellie knows if she feels she needs to see a mental health care professional or start a prescription medication, we will be by her side. The thing is, we have shifted our story, which has allowed us to make a positive impact on her life.

It can be extremely difficult to take those first steps to speak up and advocate for your child. Philippa Murphy offers several things to keep in mind:

• When going to an appointment, think about what you
  really want to tell the professional, what you'd like to know,
  and how you will ask those questions. Write them down if
  needed, so that you remember.

- If unsure of something, ask. You are not meant to know all the jargon that professionals use, and asking helps build your trust in the person who is advising you, which makes you a great advocate in choosing your trusted providers.

- Take notes. Ask how to spell things if you are unsure, and keep a good record of your appointments.

- Remember you are in charge and you should never feel pressured into choosing a path that doesn't seem right for your child. If you need more time to make decisions, then do so.[12]

When my son, Lucca, was in fifth grade, I attended his first school conference. As I sat down and got comfortable in the chair across from his teacher and his instructional assistant, I was approached with a question I didn't think I would ever have to answer again in my life.

"Do you think Lucca has ADHD?"

They both explained why they thought Lucca had ADHD and shared information about it on a piece of paper. One even said to me, "There is medication that can help."

Both women were not aware of my family's past experience with mental health. I said to them, "This has never been brought to our attention with Lucca." I continued through the conference with a lump in my throat, holding back tears. I did confirm that I would discuss it with my husband and reach out to our pediatrician with their concern.

I walked out of the building to my car, releasing my tears and reliving the emotions of my journey with Ellie. I gathered my composure and drove home. I would not allow others to dictate the direction of my son's care. They meant well, but they just didn't know our extensive experience with ADHD and the mental health system.

I followed the protocol. We visited the pediatrician, had documents sent to all his teachers to answer for his behavior, followed up with the doctor, and saw a psychologist. The psychologist didn't see anything that stood out to her as signs of ADHD, but offered to see Lucca for more appointments, giving him skills to focus in the classroom. I declined. On Lucca's medical chart, ADHD is still listed even though he was never diagnosed.

After the conference, I scheduled an appointment to speak with the school's principal to share my experience. I wanted him to know how I felt unprepared for the question from his teachers, that medications should never be implied by a school staff person, and how a teacher can't offer a diagnosis. I was advocating for my son and others like him. He is a highly sensitive boy that struggled in an overwhelming classroom. Lucca is now in high school, and I have never had anyone else bring up an issue with him and ADHD again.

WHY IS ADVOCACY SO IMPORTANT FOR THE SENSITIVE CHILD?

Supporting and nurturing our children will help them to thrive in life. Parenting a sensitive or empathic child can be difficult and a blessing all at the same time. The intensity of the emotions they feel means they're likely to become overexcited, extra angry, and super scared. Consequently, they are so focused on what other people think, they often avoid situations that might lead to embarrassment.

They might separate themselves or only have a few friends. Many have difficulty sleeping and experience nightmares. They have sensitivities to their environment, people, or animals, which can manifest as empathy. The list of blessings includes compassion, gentleness, concern about others, creativity, and intuition. The good news is that their characteristics can help change from feeling powerless and overwhelmed into capability for solving their problems. This comes from us teaching them self-advocacy.

I hope that if a child is sensitive, they have someone in their life to support them. Some of you reading this book might not be the parent; maybe you are friends or family members to this child.

Children seeking acceptance from peers and parents that don't understand what they are experiencing might choose to shut down their gifts to fit in and feel "normal." Some may even convince themselves or have family tell them that their experience is merely their imagination. Some might shut it off for self-preservation because they don't have the tools or support to use their gifts.

When children are restricted and forced to be someone they were not born to be, they start to lose confidence. Their self-worth is compromised, which causes an internal struggle with their true innate self. Internal struggles become external struggles. This is when we start to see mental illness, behavior issues, and addiction. Your child must know that they have support, as this is a part of advocacy.

Even if we don't seek the position, we find ourselves acting as advocates for our children. There is no one more motivated to see your child succeed and thrive than you!

Being an advocate for your child doesn't mean doing everything on their behalf. It means supporting them out in the world and behind the scenes as they grow into the best version of themselves. Sometimes this may look like interjecting and communicating to others for your child's best interest. Sometimes it means stepping back and supporting them quietly while they advocate for their own best solution. Listen to your child and follow their needs, helping them, validating them, and of course loving them.

It can be hard to think clearly when you're in a crisis. You may hear conflicting advice from family, friends, partners, doctors, psychiatrists, or even yourself. Let your intuition help guide you back on track.

Intuition can come through as a knowing, a gut feeling, an aha moment, or a dream. Intuition allows you to go with the flow and trust your inner voice to guide you toward advocating for something important. When you advocate for yourself or your child, you do so because you want to see change, educate people, make a difference, and raise awareness.

HOW TO HELP YOUR CHILD ADVOCATE FOR THEMSELVES

Part of being an effective advocate is teaching our children to advocate for themselves, because we won't always be by their side for guidance. Part of taking care of your child is teaching the powerful skill of self-advocacy. For children, self-advocacy is when they understand their strengths and weaknesses, know what they need to succeed, and are able to communicate these needs to other people. That is not a natural skill for some, so it takes practice and support from their parents.

Ellie has learned to speak up and advocate for herself. She didn't want to return to public school for ninth grade. She knew in her gut that it wouldn't be a good fit for her. If we even drove near the school, she had an emotional and physical reaction. She sought out opportunities for education through an online school. Her father and I weren't sure this would be a good option, so we told her she had to provide us with information and share why she wanted to attend an online school. She did her research and explained clearly why it would be better for her to participate in online school than public school. We accepted her reasoning, and she attended an online school from ninth to twelfth grade. It wasn't easy, but her mental and emotional health improved so much because she advocated for herself and her needs. Ellie graduated from the online high school in 2018.

According to Andrew M. I. Lee, "Self-advocacy can be broken down into a few key elements." He shares a few:

• Understanding specific needs. (This is part of self-awareness.)

• Knowing what help or support will address those needs, like tutoring or a classroom setting.

• Communicating those needs to teachers and others.

Here are some ways to help your child develop self-advocacy:

• Talk with your child about strengths and weaknesses.

• Remind your child that asking for help is a good thing.

• Praise your child's efforts of speaking up.

• Encourage your child to use classroom accommodations.

• When a problem comes up, give your child a chance to solve it before stepping in.

• Let your child have a say in decisions about school.[13]

Many people don't talk or share when their child experiences differences, whether they are spiritual, emotional, mental, or physical. We did not for many years. It could be due to fear of judgment, stigma, or denial. Being in this space didn't allow us to be open advocates for Ellie. We weren't great examples of sharing her true self with others. This disempowered her to ask for help or advocate for herself.

Don't be afraid of having your voice heard or your words read. Our personal experience is evidence that there are real emotions and people behind the story, allowing for empathy. Empathy allows you to challenge someone's emotional attachment to a belief so you can move their support toward your perspective. Sharing what has or hasn't worked for your family is like an invitation for others to share. There is a power that exists in being vulnerable, and it comes from being authentic.

It took me years of healing to be able to share our journey. If you do not share in a safe space, this could validate your child's feelings of being different. This can lead to guilt and loneliness. As parents, we need to be informed and advocate for our children. Searching out or creating support groups is so important. Learn more in a future chapter about building community.

Chapter Nine

HOLISTIC HEALTH PATHWAYS

y mother-in-law bought Ellie the book *I Think, I Am!*
Teaching Kids the Power of Affirmations by Louise Hay
and Kristina Tracy when she was ten years old. She
found the book at a gift shop and thought it would be a fun and
supportive read for Ellie. It was colorful, with images of children
in everyday situations, and gave examples of how they control their
thoughts. I had no clue who Louise Hay was or that she spent her
life's work teaching people how to live a positive and empowered
life with positive statements, which she called affirmations. The
book was fun and colorful. I read it a few times with Ellie, and
then it was placed on her bookshelf in her room.

Years later, when I started to search out healing for myself, I
stumbled upon Louise Hay, who taught that our emotions and
thoughts are energy and if they are not expressed "in motion," they
can become stuck in the body. It was a new concept to me. I found
it interesting, and I purchased her book *You Can Heal Your Life*.
This book was a simple read but very impactful on my outlook of
how we treat ourselves and our self-worth. The book mentions
how our limiting beliefs can create disease or illness and how if
you change your thoughts, you can change your life. I felt this was
something I could do. I was already an optimist, but I needed to
shift my negative thoughts about myself using daily affirmations.
This also reminded me of the children's book on Ellie's bookshelf.
Was it a coincidence? Or was this children's book divinely placed
in our lives to validate a shift in thinking? I had a moment of

enlightenment. We supported Ellie in other ways even before we were aware of the importance of alternative healing approaches.

FOOD AND THE SENSITIVE

A common way to fill an emotional void or lack of acceptance is with food. Some foods release hormones in your brain—endorphins and dopamine. Both are feel-good hormones. Ellie's eating habits changed when she was first prescribed medication for anxiety. She enjoyed the high fats, carbohydrates, and sugar found in sweets, pasta, pizza, snacks, and fast food.

After school, Ellie demanded fast food. "I want McDonald's," she said, day in and day out. I gave in to her, knowing she had a tough day at school, and I also didn't want to upset her by saying no. She was relentless in asking, crying, or yelling to get what she wanted, and though I did say no at times, I eventually gave in to her requests. This was almost every day after school, from third until sixth grade, and represented a common theme in our relationship.

Giving in is about you, not your child. It is your lack of knowing who you are as a parent and person. It's wanting to comfort your child and not feel like a bad parent. Personally, my fear of disappointing Ellie came from my relationship with my own mother, a never-ending give and take of myself. I didn't want to upset, so I needed to be what others wanted me to be. But who was I? Who should I be for my daughter? I had been a chameleon for most of my life, and found I couldn't answer those questions. But by giving in to Ellie, I was not being the parent she needed me to be. I knew it was wrong, but didn't know how to stop. Breaking the pattern seemed scary and overwhelming to me. It was easiest to continue and not shake the boat. I wasn't ready or strong enough for that journey yet.

I was feeding my dog a high-quality and more nutritional diet than my daughter. We fostered dogs for many years, and it was essential to the rescue group that we supply the dogs with the highest quality diet. Yet I fed my own child a poor-quality diet of fast food, sugar, and few fruits and vegetables. My connection to my daughter was based on her emotional need versus her physical need to be healthy.

Going back to the book by Louise Hay, *You Can Heal Your Life*, I was not allowing for my daughter to heal her life or even create a space for living a healthy life. I started to research the link between processed foods and mental health, and realized the impact food was playing on Ellie's behavior and mood.

It wasn't until I became aware that these unhealthy habits could contribute to mental health in a highly sensitive person that I began to limit her processed foods. This was not without push-back from Ellie. Sugary fast foods are addictive, and our emotions can get in the way of making change. We made the shift slowly by not entirely eliminating but limiting the amounts she ate. I was so interested in supporting other families in eating healthy that I became certified as a kids' nutrition specialist.

At the age of twelve, Ellie was diagnosed with binge eating after completing an eating disorder assessment at The Emily Program. We didn't follow through with their outpatient treatment suggestions because we were still dealing with her mental health struggles with other care providers.

Years later, after realizing Ellie was a sensitive empath, I found more information by Dr. Judith Orloff about empaths and binge eating. Overeating and food addictions are common among empaths. She writes, "Frequently, the specific addiction is to sugar or carbohydrates."[14] The empath often experiences binge eating and weight gain when faced with ongoing stressful situations because of their body's reaction to the negative energy in the environment around them. The negative energy stimulates the hunger response in their brain as their body attempts to shield itself by adding a layer of fat as protection from the toxicity.

This all makes sense with Ellie. She felt the emotional overload from school, which was causing her stress, and as a result, she would binge eat. She was blocking out her sensitivity and the fact that she was not being understood or accepted as her true self. Food was one of her coping mechanisms, just like her mother.

ANIMALS AND SENSITIVES

Horses are highly attuned to environmental activity and sensitive to people's emotional states. They react instinctively to your attitude and your signals. Horses are also very caring creatures. They are an amazing form of therapy, especially for animal lovers like Ellie. When one of her therapists mentioned horseback riding and its positive benefits on emotional well-being, we felt this was a fun way to support Ellie. I found a local barn that had openings for lessons. Ellie and I drove about thirty minutes south of our house in the city to a rural community. Ellie was apprehensive to step out of the car but slowly came out and walked behind me. We knocked on the office door to be greeted by a teenaged girl named Jordy, who gave Ellie and me a tour of the barn, introduced us to some of the horses, and explained the lesson plan. I could see the excitement in Ellie's face even if she didn't want to speak. We thanked Jordy for her time and walked to our car. I asked Ellie what she thought, and she responded, "I want lessons."

Ellie's lessons included grooming and preparing the horse to ride, learning the horse's personality, learning proper form, and additional care. These times took her away from her thoughts. She was so focused on the lesson at hand. She took lessons for about one year and then wanted to quit. Missing her time with horses, she returned to lessons when she was seventeen and continued for almost a year until the barn closed. We searched out a new barn, but we never found one that felt good to Ellie.

Ellie loves animals of all kinds. Growing up, I always had a dog. My husband never had a pet until I came along. When Ellie was five years old, we got a dog, Raleigh, who needed a home because his owner was moving into an apartment. I convinced my husband to bring this dog into our home. He was a big black Lab, full of love and energy.

Years later, we fostered dogs with an excellent local rescue group called Underdog Rescue, founded by a friend of mine from high school. I thought we could give it a try, and my husband agreed, not knowing this would end up being a four-year experience. Many of the dogs were from puppy mills and were used for breeding. They spent their lives in a metal cage, never seeing daylight or running in a yard.

We brought them into our home and gave them the love they had never known. We made sure they had a wonderful family to go to after their time with ours, where they learned to be regular dogs. This showed my children that you can love and release. We were fosters when Ellie was in elementary school during the beginning of her mental illness journey. At that time, it was especially important for all of us to watch a dog transition from a skittish, scared animal to trusting and flourishing. Fostering takes patience, love, and a good eye for observation, which we had.

We moved to a new home in 2018. We found the perfect house on a quiet cul-de-sac, with a pond in the backyard and woods across the street.

"Mom, we live in the country now," my son remarked when we moved in. He was used to a busier environment, like our old home in the city. This was the perfect home for a sensitive empath, where we could have a deep connection with both nature and animals.

The health benefits of spending time in nature and being around animals are well known. Whether it's hiking with our dog, riding a horse, or birdwatching, time spent in nature remedies the overload, stress, and anxiety we often experience.

Animals have a lot to teach us. Animals embody natural tendencies to love and trust others. They teach us things like acceptance, resilience, and living in the present moment.

ALWAYS SEARCHING

Even before making the giant leap to a holistic approach to mental health, I searched and tried to improve Ellie's mental well-being congruent with her mental health care providers. Our journey is and has always been about balancing the different ways to support Ellie. The balance is developing the tools that work for you or your child. You don't have to be all or nothing when it comes to the care of yourself or others. Find what works best for you and your family.

After I purchased that first simple tool from a local women's store and began to see positive changes in my child, I recalled the small steps I had already taken toward supporting Ellie. These alternative ideas were enough to move forward in the space of holistic modalities. This was an *aha* moment! The right people were coming into my life for a reason, sharing a message I needed to receive at that moment. When you see your child change for the better, it gives you hope. No matter if it was a mental or energic shift, it was happening. We had tried the traditional route for so many years, and nothing was better until we stopped.

Whatever the cause, the effect is what we cared about. I started to look at Ellie's mental illness and challenges as characteristics of an empathic and gifted child. This might seem like a quick shift from traditional medicine to a holistic path, but we had seen our child struggle daily for years, and we were all ready to make any change that would be beneficial to Ellie. There were two overarching ways I made the decision to shift her care. The first was my research for other possible factors or causes of mental illness.

The second was listening inwardly to my intuition. I believe my intuition working in concert with complex information led to better decision-making. Intuition exists in all of us, whether we acknowledge it or not. Understanding it can give you great insights into your own mind, and thus how to use it to improve your life.

As I embarked on this new path, which brought us to look at mental illness from a different perspective, I realized the lack of resources and information available to support families. I am here to provide support and knowledge to others. This is my family's truth, and I share it so you know there is another way. We are now seven-plus years on this different path. I do not dispute the value of traditional medicine in some cases. I embrace a health care model that emphasizes the power of mind, body, and spirit in healing and general well-being.

I am a person who needs awareness to move forward. Just like when Ellie received her first diagnosis, I had something to explain the behavior, and I was able to move forward, even though it was challenging. If I have awareness around chaos, then I can accept and move forward. It is the unknown that causes me to stress.

After stumbling through the darkness, we must learn to walk in the light. We search for meaning and try to bring our lives into focus. Sometimes we struggle with the lack of clarity and purpose in our lives. If you're looking to change the world, start by improving yourself. Have a better understanding of who you are by learning from your challenges. If you want to find inner peace in life, the first step is to accept yourself for who you are. The second step is to stop comparing yourself to others. Once you do this, it's much easier to accept other people for who they are.

To ask society to shift their perspective and ideas is challenging, but you create a ripple effect of change in others when you improve yourself. You might think you cannot change the world canvas, but you can. I know this truth from personal experience. I took Ellie for her annual physical, and the nurse asked the usual questions. She was going over the list of medications that were on the computer for Ellie. For each one—except the list of vitamins—I kept saying, "She no longer takes that."

The nurse paused and asked me about the antidepressant prescription Ellie was no longer taking. "I'm currently on the same one," she confided, "but I've still been experiencing depression."

I told the nurse I believed specific medication had increased Ellie's depression and suicidal ideation. I also recommended the nurse speak with her doctor. My kindness—my essence—allowed the nurse to feel comfortable with me to open and share private information. I thanked her for sharing with me her struggle with the same prescription. This is just one example of making an impact on someone's life.

Small actions can become real. Significant steps just get lost to fear and inaction. The challenge of shifting society is like building a bridge to connect one side to another. The challenge is finding ways to connect people who are disconnected by their own beliefs, and the complexity is in making it happen. We all have our own beliefs, and changing those can be challenging. It is not our responsibility to change everyone's beliefs, but we can give them a glimpse of awareness to another perspective on giftedness, mental illness, education, medical care, and holistic care.

Creating a bridge between our medical system and holistic therapies would be amazing. This is starting to happen. Reiki, a specific form of energy healing, "is beginning to gain acceptance at hospitals and clinics across America as a meaningful and cost-effective way to improve patient care."[15] In addition, "aromatherapy and essential oils have been introduced into hospital settings over the last few years to benefit patients, relatives, and hospital staff."[16]

BE MINDFUL

We were told by Ellie's therapist to thank our daughter for clearing the dinner table. We thought this was ridiculous as she should do this chore without being given praise. But we tried it. It felt awkward at first saying, "Thank you for clearing the dinner table," or, "Thank you for doing the dishes."

What we learned was that giving praise was planting a seed of resilience. We had to step out of our ego or idea of when we would give credit and allow her to feel a sense of accomplishment to build on her confidence. This is also us being mindful by showing Ellie how we valued her. Don't focus on what your child "should" do or be, but instead, notice what is already there.

This continued as I learned to understand Ellie for her true self, a sensitive empath, a fantastic reader, a gamer, a kind and generous person, a wise soul, and a bright light. Slowly, I stopped trying to push her into someone she was not meant to be. Once I allowed her this space, she could be open to who she was and experience her life authentically, and not as a reaction to what others wanted her to be.

I started to pay more attention to being present in the moment. This required slowing down my thoughts and paying attention to what was happening in the present without changing anything. Being mindful helped me acknowledge different feelings and emotions rather than push them away. When we are mindful, we accept ourselves just as we are without judgment. I started to practice meditation daily to quiet my mind and build a skill of responding to situations with intention rather than an impulsive knee-jerk reaction. When my mind is quiet, I can tap into my intuition, which provides a space for better insight and choices.

I provided Ellie a space to speak up about discontinuing her prescription medications. I focused on being mindful, and pausing instead of reacting. This was probably one of the most critical moments when she felt truly heard because I didn't interrupt or respond quickly. I was calm about what I believed would be the next step, speaking with her father. I didn't know that during the time between the question and the decision I would meet a woman at a meeting who would present clarity. Receiving clarity and listening to my intuition sparked the next direction on our journey.

MEETING SPIRITUAL TEACHERS

I was so lucky to attract amazing women into my networking group—they were the women I needed at that time of my life. Some attended a meeting but never joined, but all were brought to me for a reason. The law of attraction is a simple idea: we attract what we project.

One of these amazing women was Nicole, a Reiki master and shaman working at a local wellness center. Nicole was gently pressured to attended one of my meetings by a coworker. I could tell by her gentle presence that she was someone I wanted to know better. I had no idea what a Reiki master did or what energy healing meant, but I felt she was the one to learn from. I started to see Nicole for energy healing sessions to help me release trauma, emotional and mental stress, and other blocks to my personal growth stored in my body's energy fields.

Reiki is a Japanese technique for energy healing in which a practitioner places his or her hands on or just above the patient's body to channel universal life energy, promoting harmony and balance. I see my Reiki master about every three months or more if I feel the need. It keeps me feeling like I am in flow and balance. Ellie has also seen Nicole, and said the healing sessions were more helpful than therapy. She didn't have to speak, just lie on the table while Nicole worked to clear blocks and rebalance her energy.

Nicole brought my attention to shadow work and past life regression. I didn't realize I was doing shadow work when I started my healing journey. I didn't have a name for the deep dive I took into the darker aspect of myself. As a child I didn't feel I could fully express myself to my family or friends. I was an only child for twelve years and felt a sense of loneliness and disconnection from others. My mom cared for me when I was ill and made meals, but I never felt a deep bond like my mom had with her mom, and I couldn't comprehend why we didn't have that relationship. Empaths find it challenging to be around others who are not genuine. They need honest, deep, meaningful relationships. If someone's emotions don't meet what they are expressing, it creates a disconnect for the empath and a lack of trust.

The "shadow" is a concept first coined by Swiss psychiatrist Carl Jung that describes those aspects of the personality that we choose to reject and repress. For one reason or another, we all have parts of ourselves that we don't like—or that we think society won't like—so we push those parts down into our unconscious psyches. It is this collection of repressed aspects of our identity that Jung referred to as our "shadow self."

When we were children, our brain was like a sponge, absorbing all the emotions that were flowing through us. If we experienced fear, anger, shame, or sadness, those negative emotions impacted our brain and had a lasting effect on how we perceive ourselves and interact with others. By embracing our shadow sides, we can live from a place of strength and love. If we ignore these parts of ourselves, they tend to fester and poison our lives.

Through shadow work, we can begin to heal those early wounds to live a fuller life. Shadow work involves facing and integrating the less desirable parts of ourselves and digging deeper into who we really are.

My shadow self creeps in around my self-esteem. I used to fill this space with clothes, the newest and greatest toys, or cars, thinking others would like me because of those material things, and in turn, I would like myself. I also worked hard to be a good girl and not cause any disappointment for my parents or friends. This left me feeling restrained, non-expressive, and like a conformist. I rejected important parts of myself, which manifested in pushing down the pain with food and poor spending habits.

Many are resistant to shadow work. For me, it has truly been a beautiful space to heal and understand who I am and what I need. We stuff our traumas way down deep in the psyche. In other words, the bad things that happen to you (especially at young ages) leave permanent imprints. They create fears, beliefs, and tendencies in us that we forget about. Shadow work cultivates self-compassion and self-awareness. I did this through journaling, meditation, and self-love practices.

Further on in my healing journey, I had a past life regression session with Nicole. I was curious to see who I was in a past life and if it brought clarity to my current life. I was put into a meditative state, or light hypnosis. I lay on her table just as I did with Reiki. She calmly talked through possible past life experiences. Once I stepped into my awareness of a past life, she asked non-leading questions aloud and wrote down my answers for my own record. After this experience, I could see patterns in my current life and past life. I was a Native American elder holding a circle with women and children in that past life. That circle was still my mission now, and I became able to understand this on a deeper level from this experience with Nicole.

When you embrace new experiences and don't fear them, they will embrace you back with new opportunities to grow. Years later, I held monthly empowerment circles at the metaphysical center. I once walked into that space as an unsure mom attending a drumming circle, and now I was a spiritual teacher. I became aware of different modalities and tools that worked for me to heal. I introduced Ellie to options and opportunities for her to develop her own tools. I also allowed her the space to choose her own path to healing, not pushing her in any direction but creating her journey and embracing her as Ellie.

HIGHER VIBRATION

Over time I learned self-compassion for my journey and for others. Compassion is an expression of support and an act of empathy. When you have compassion or feel empathy for someone, it's important to acknowledge their feelings without trying to change them.

When we struggled with Ellie's mental illness journey, our family lived from a lower vibrational state like sadness and overwhelm. Illness, disease, and troubling emotions are usually associated with low or unbalanced vibration or energy flow. Our family was living from a disempowered state, leaving us to experience daily stress, loss of control, and uncertainty. Disempowering thoughts can create negative emotions, poor health, lack of spiritual connection, anxiety, anger, fear, jealousy, or feeling stuck. We were giving our power away to others, and feeling like passengers rather than driving our daughter's care, until we were ready to take control of the situation and turn toward a different path.

When you are on a healing journey, even small changes can have a considerable impact. Once I worked on self-understanding and felt empowering thoughts, positive emotions, good health, and solid spiritual connections, things lined up for me. The law of attraction says, "Like attracts Like," meaning the frequency of what we put out into the world will always reflect back to us.

CREATING MY OWN PRACTICES

Over the years I spent learning and applying different techniques and tools to support my transformation, I created a practice that works for me. From my experience, healing is most effective in a multilayered approach. I combined many different techniques along my journey. Some I still use, and some didn't work or feel right to me. Drumming, for example, is not something I currently practice, but maybe I will return to it someday. Similarly, I found a healer, Nicole, whose practices work for me, as opposed to other healers with other styles—like Jessica, who first saw Ellie for a session—that may work better for another.

I have a morning ritual that includes meditation, journaling, and a card pull from either an oracle or angel card deck. I set an intention for my day and say an affirmation. This is not what my life was like before my awakening. I never used words like intention or ritual. I didn't carry crystals in my pocket or spray essential oils before leaving the house.

It took me stepping out of my comfort zone as an introverted sensitive empath to try new things. Stepping out of your comfort zone can be scary, and I know it was for me. This is understandable. Since we were children, we have been taught that pain, discomfort, and fear are bad for us, or a sign we have done something wrong. But if we overcome that discomfort, we can do anything. We can temporarily leave our old identity behind and go through a period of self-growth. Who we are today is not who we were yesterday. Who we will be tomorrow is not who we are today. Beliefs and attitudes change over time, and that change is a necessary part of life.

DUALITY AND THE SENSITIVE EMPATH

Ellie's struggle with anxiety and depression meant there was a lot of darkness before the light of coming off prescription medication. Once she was able to find love and understanding of herself as a sensitive empath, she was open to self-discovery and healing. Being an empath is often considered a blessing and a curse, though I prefer to say "challenge" instead of "curse." One of the challenges is that the depth of our feelings can develop physical and emotional symptoms. Many of us struggle with people-pleasing and poor boundaries. The blessing is empathizing deeply. We are very intuitive and skilled at reading people, circumstances, and situations more than others. We are renowned as natural healers, creatives, and deep thinkers.

Unless you know that you are a sensitive empath you may find life to be challenging, or even experience a mental health problem. Being a sensitive empath brings great awareness of the emotions of others, which can make us vulnerable to anxiety and depression. For highly sensitive children, too much emotional and physical stimuli can cause them to behave erratically and even develop behavioral problems. So, they are often medicated. This ongoing pressure to be "normal"—whatever that is—often leads to a culture of kids medicated for their "behaviors." This is an example of how society sees some children as normal versus different. When we don't understand their differences, it creates a much more significant problem. It causes a lack of self-acceptance that often continues into adulthood.

If you're a sensitive empath, chances are you've had to hide your true self, which caused you to feel isolated and misunderstood. That's why it's important to spend time learning about what it means to be a sensitive empath. Don't hide in a world of duality, where you pretend to be something you're not. Instead, live in the present moment fully and be yourself. When you live from that place, you can teach your children to do the same.

Our society is filled with duality—good and evil, right and wrong, beautiful and ugly. But while this division exists in so many aspects of life, you can still find harmony and balance in your own life. I am someone who feels like they live in the in-between, a space between two contrasting conditions, creating a balance. My balance falls between the realms of spiritual/religious, mainstream/holistic, intuitive/logical, and strong/weak, to name a few. We live in a world of extremes. It can feel bold to live your life in the in-between. Some might think that this is the easy way out. I embrace this space by creating my own experiences based on my needs and intuition.

I no longer want to be the chameleon who mirrors other people's actions or emotions. I strive for alignment with who I am and choose to create the world where I want to live. Embrace your inbetweenness! I believe in the importance of balancing mainstream and traditional medicine, and found life-changing transformation in holistic or alternative modalities. I call myself a Catholic, and I also use spiritual practices that support me. No more being a chameleon, adjusting myself to be what others want me to be. I can choose how I show up and who I allow into my life. I believe in creating what is best for you. As I share our journey, I hope you take what feels right to you intuitively and leave the rest. Create your own healing journey.

Becoming aware of your personal power and choosing to be a healthy, sensitive empath has everything to do with how you perceive yourself and the world around you.

INTUITION

Have you ever experienced a time when you just knew something was off? Maybe you were driving home from work, and you had a feeling you should take a different road, so you did and later found out an accident occurred where you usually would have been driving. I am sure you can think of many examples when tuning in to your intuition—or ignoring it—produced a notable outcome. I shared some of my experiences with you, from meeting certain people to starting a networking group and attending a specific class. Your intuition is the compass guiding you toward greatness. Dr. Seymour Epstein said, "Intuition involves a sense of knowing without knowing how one knows."

I felt connected to my growing intuition as I experienced my awakening. I learned to listen to, rather than ignore, the guidance of my intuition. This is your voice of your soul. It is not easy to listen to your innermost self. First, you need to recognize who you are, to discern clearly what is your own voice, untangled from the multitude of confusing voices inside you from others, past and present. Listening to yourself and your inner voice is a skill that can be acquired through self-reflection, meditation, and self-knowledge.

It does take courage to trust yourself and rely on your own instincts. As a culture, we have learned that we should look at things logically. There seems to be high value placed on logic or reasoning. We need to use both our head and heart. This is listening to all aspects of ourselves, which help us gain a more complete view of life.

Trusting and believing in your own intuition, without needing to justify or defend it, is part of becoming a person with your own opinions and ways of thinking. I came to this point as we traveled the path of Ellie's mental illness. I began to be open to my intuition and followed what I felt was next with our journey.

Growing up, I was taught the power of thought, logic, and reasoning. Schools teach us the basics, but they neglect emotional intelligence. I don't ever remember being taught about intuition or listening to my feelings. Instead of speaking up, I often suppressed what I felt in order to go along with others and blend in.

Ellie's experience with stomachaches and headaches in elementary school, being diagnosed with opposition defiant disorder, and in middle school having a conversation brought up about her possibly experiencing dissociation are symptoms I believe came from the lack of connection to her knowing. As an intuitive young woman, she is a deep thinker and can be absorbed in her own world. Everyday life felt pointless, dull, and boring, which showed up as depression. And anxiety showed up because she wasn't connected to the now or present. She was focused on the "what ifs" and the future.

When she experienced a stomachache, she was told she was alright, but Ellie knew something was wrong. I listened to Ellie, but then I would try to fix what was causing her pain instead of allowing her to feel the pain and learn from the feeling. I should have let her share and express her feelings with no action but love from me. My mistake came from never letting her strengthen her intuition by personal experience.

Talk with your child about events when they may have ignored their intuition and let them know how important it is to listen. Keeping kids focused on self-talk and feeling recognition will help them center their voice, reduce self-doubt, and maintain interpersonal boundaries. With our help, children learn that they have feelings that guide their behavior, and that their feelings reflect their needs, wants, and beliefs. When I began to share how I felt and used my intuition as a guide, it opened the space for Ellie to do the same. Start by shutting off your inner critic who needs to rationalize everything and just listen—*without* judgment. You must first be willing to hear the truth in your heart. Keep a journal or a dream journal or start a synchronicity notebook to write down all your so-called coincidences. Start simply following your hunches and prepare to be amazed by where they lead you.

Chapter Ten

CREATING A FAMILY SUPPORT SYSTEM

Going through a challenging journey with Ellie taught me to be compassionate with myself. Being able to forgive yourself requires empathy, compassion, kindness, and understanding. It also requires the knowledge that forgiveness is a choice. I could sit in the darkness and be hard on myself and others for the turmoil we experienced, but how would that serve anyone? I came to a place where I had to forgive myself for all decisions I made in the past. I was doing what I thought was best for my child at that time. It was through my healing process that I was able to understand the most important person to show compassion to was me. I already have a strong compassion for others but was lacking it for myself.

When practicing self-compassion, we transform shame. When we are in shame, it is a signal that we are out of alignment with our true self and values. Self-compassion allows you a starting place to flourish not just personally but in your relationships. Self-compassion encourages you to know your most uncomfortable parts and create a more peaceful existence, as you approach whatever you experienced as shameful with curiosity and kindness. As Mahatma Gandhi said, "You must be the change you want to see in the world."

Compassion is the driving force behind social connections. It's what leads parents to meet the ever-demanding needs of their children. It plays a strong role in relationships between adults, too.

Compassion leads us to act on behalf of our friends and loved ones, to do those little things that strengthen our connections. Compassion is what causes us to want to do something in the aftermath of disasters or tragic events.

Empathy is what makes us human. It helps us to relate with others and see things from their perspective. This connection enables us to understand why people make certain decisions and connect more deeply.

Empathy and compassion force us to look beyond ourselves and broaden our perspectives. Reaching out to others in need builds social connections and enhances the interpersonal skills necessary for healthy relationships. It demonstrates care and allows us to show our authentic selves.

Our relationships with others can be both the most joyful and most challenging aspects of our lives. We learn a lot about ourselves from our relationships with others. I learned to be more understanding of myself and others from my daughter. I learned compassion from my husband, especially when facing difficult times as a family. And I learned humor from my son. A sense of humor helps relieve stress.

USING COMPASSION IN YOUR FAMILY

- Allow yourself to feel negative emotions without judging them as "bad" or "wrong." If you do this, you will feel less stressed and more in control.

- If you and your spouse have different approaches to handling challenges and obstacles, you can combine your strengths and overcome your weaknesses. Be ready to compromise, listen, and be open to new ideas.

- There is power in words. I found it helpful to use daily affirmations and reframe my negative thoughts into positive ones to elevate my mood.

- Create a self-care practice to reduce stress and protect your well-being as a parent.

- Be present for your other children. When one child struggles, we tend to focus on that child, so carve out time to focus on your other kids. They might be hurting too.

- What I have heard from other moms is that they are ready to shift and see their child differently, but their spouse is not in the same place. I used my mother's intuition to do what was best for my child and hoped that my husband had trust and support in my decisions. I saw our daughter's spiritual gifts and he wasn't ready or open. I needed to keep moving forward for the best interest of our daughter. He never told me what to do or not do, because he had trust in me. He saw the change in her and knew whatever I was doing was working and supported the change.

- Self-understanding and healing create a healthier, happier, and more positive environment for the whole family.

Within the dynamics of our family, we all have different roles and functions. These various roles can come about because of how our family dynamics play out or our own individual choices and personalities. When you have a family member with any type of struggle or medical issue, this may distract the family dynamic, and can make for a challenging time for the entire family.

If you have other children, they may be jealous if you focus all the attention on their sibling's mental health challenges. Time, attention, and resources are often compromised as the family responds to symptoms and seeks treatment and support. Additionally, they are witnessing their sibling's struggle, which can be an emotionally challenging experience.

My son was only two years old when Ellie was first diagnosed. He grew up not knowing anything different. Going to appointments and seeing her act out was his norm. As he got older and more aware of Ellie's negative behavior, he often did the opposite and acted especially good. He would even bring attention to himself by saying, "Look at me, Mom, I am good." Lucca could see how upset I got with his sister and he didn't want to upset me in the same way. I didn't want him to take on the role of "good child," so I made sure to explain to him that Ellie wasn't bad, she was showing bad behavior or making a bad decision.

Lucca did ask at one point, "Why does Ellie act so bad?" We sat down with him and explained that his sister had an illness that made her brain have trouble with certain things and caused her to react in a certain way. When she went to the doctor, we told him, they were helping her feel better.

Just recently, Lucca told me that he thought his sister went to jail when he was little. Now, we can laugh about it because he knows Ellie wasn't in jail, but it brought up how a little child doesn't understand when a family member is struggling with mental illness and goes away to a facility. Children will use a relatable image to create their own story.

Families need strong, healthy communication to function well and meet the individual needs of all family members. Communication happens whether families work at it or allow it to happen. Even if you don't talk, you are communicating with nonverbal language. Sensitives can pick up on the energy of others in a room without anyone speaking.

FIVE-TIER APPROACH

Find a way for your family to come together to support your sensitive or empathic child, your other child, your relationship with your spouse or significant other, family unit, and yourself. When you are in sync in your relationships, you can grow and expand in love. This is not easy. It takes time, support, and focus.

1. You and the Sensitive Child

When Ellie was in seventh grade sitting in the lunchroom with friends, someone threw an apple, and it hit her on the back. This might not be a big deal to some kids, but it was extremely upsetting to a sensitive child. I share this story because I want to convey to you that a situation that might seem small to one child can be a form of trauma to a sensitive child. Trauma of any level carries forward in life if not resolved. Minor traumas are situations that make an impact on us but don't include things like death, physical injury, or sexual violence. According to The Substance Abuse and Mental Health Services Association (SAMHSA), "Trauma is an event or series of events that is experienced as physically or emotionally threatening and that has lasting adverse effects on the individual's functioning." That means trauma can be different for each person. We could experience the same exact situation and walk away from that experience with completely different emotional and mental perspectives.

Trauma can impact our lives in different ways. Ellie had feelings of unworthiness and could feel the aggression behind that incident. Other situations in that school caused her to have physical feelings when we would drive by, and for years, she didn't even want to enter the building.

We didn't realize at the time how upsetting some of the experiences Ellie had were to her and how they would affect her long term. As we became aware of her empathic and sensitive feelings, we realized she needed to be parented differently. She didn't respond well to authoritative discipline or more assertive action on our part. According to Dr. Elaine Aron, "The authoritarian parent provides an excess of structure and fails to balance it with communication, explanation, or discussion. They may degrade the child, ignore his or her experience, or violate a young one's need to feel safe in their own home. This produces fear, resentment, low self-esteem, a risk of counter-aggression, and perhaps later rebellion against various forms of authority. The parents believe obedience equals love when actually it indicates submissiveness, not affection." This was more of my husband's type of parenting.

My type of parenting was permissive, which Dr. Aron describes as follows: "This form of lenient, non-confrontational, indulgent parenting is beneficial in that parents are nurturing and loving. But rules are often too flexible or are never articulated. Children may need to be bribed with outsized rewards to cooperate. This produces children who may be self-absorbed and have difficulty sharing. In school, their performance may be lackadaisical. They may be unwilling to conform to reasonable directions from teachers. As a teen and an adult, they may be surprised by the consequence's life imposes on their ill-considered actions."

Our parenting types combined created a confusing and anxious environment for a sensitive child. Ellie needed to be given limitations and calm interaction. We didn't start to parent this way until after she came home from the inpatient residential treatment facility. There were times I had to remind my husband to talk with her in a different tone or how to approach her when he was upset. This made a huge difference in our relationship with Ellie. She felt respected and heard, but still with boundaries and discipline.

The sensitive child can be a handful when they're young and may need to be parented differently to enable them to function and succeed as adults. This didn't become clear to me until after experiencing our struggles with Ellie's mental illness. These children are often self-motivated and inner-directed, and they are persistent. As parents we need to resist the impulse to "break their will," because strong-willed kids often become leaders and changemakers.

How to Practice Awareness and Empathy with Your Highly Sensitive Child

- Listen. Sometimes they don't need advice, they just need you to listen.

- Recognize what triggers cause your child to feel overwhelmed and overstimulated. Being more aware of the stressors in your child's environment can help you better prepare your child.

- Be responsive. It's easy to tell your child to get over it, or to calm down. Unfortunately, reacting that way may just make the matter worse. Instead, acknowledge what's happening without giving the situation too much attention.

- Focus on strengths. Praise your child for the activities where they shine. Don't compare them to other children.

- Create a calm area. Provide a special space for them for when they feel overwhelmed or upset. They can help by putting items they enjoy in the space, like books, blankets, stuffed animals, or drawing materials.

- Set clear boundaries. Our children need parents who are consistent, clear, and healthy. They need boundaries that are clear yet forgiving enough to encourage their development.

2. You and Your Other Children

My son, Lucca, is six years younger than my daughter.

When he asked me, "Why is Ellie so mean?" he was only four or five years old, but was well-accustomed to seeing his sister be aggressive and angry in our home. He had even been a trigger or target for his sister's outbursts. I had to explain to him that she had an illness that caused her to behave in this way and that she saw a doctor to receive care. Living with a sibling that has a mental illness can be difficult. They may be treated differently, and they may have a hard time coping with what's going on. Others may not want to burden their parents with their problems.

It was important to me to be there for my son. I was very aware of how Ellie's issues could be affecting Lucca in the moment and the future. I made myself available for questions he had or any emotions he was experiencing, giving him my full attention when needed. As parents, we never blamed Ellie for her experiences. Lucca is a more reserved and laid-back child. We never felt the need to seek out professional help for Lucca, though it is an option if needed at any time, as you never know when these old stories will show up in his life.

All children have a different temperament. Temperament is something we're born with—it's a set of traits that makes each of us unique, and it's an influential factor in determining how we react to the world. The way a child approaches a new situation is one example of temperament. My son is calm and laid back. He's a say-it-how-he-sees-it kind of kid. The very opposite of his sister. I believe God gave him to me on purpose so I didn't completely lose my mind. It is important to gauge each child's unique temperament and parent to that specific child.

When you have more than one child you also gain experience raising children, but each child has their own style and needs. Most parents seem to be more confident after their first child. For me, I felt less anxious to care for my son. Plus, my children were six years apart. I didn't have to care for two little ones at the same time.

Lucca loved his sister but didn't understand why she acted so mean to him at times. We had a pool in our backyard. One of our turning points was when Ellie held him underwater, and I was watching from the kitchen window. I ran out to the porch yelling, "Let him up!" He was scared and crying. This was one of the moments when we felt our son was no longer safe with his sister, and it added to our decision to send her for treatment.

Supporting your sensitive child's sibling(s) is so important. Don't let them get pushed aside or lost in the urgency of the other child's needs. Depending on their age, they might not understand what is happening and why, or they might be very aware but need an explanation and guidance from you or a therapist.

How to Help Your Mentally-Ill Child's Sibling

- If you have other children, it's important to provide time and resources for them. Having a happy and balanced family can make it easier for everyone to handle stress.

- Provide a family culture of understanding and allow your child to express love or support for their mentally ill sibling in appropriate ways.

- Listen to their questions and concerns about their sibling. Answer the best you can in an age-appropriate manner.

- When speaking with siblings, foster a sense of hope.

- Support their efforts to learn more about their sibling's diagnosis.

• You may even encourage them to seek professional help to better understand their sibling and their own experiences.

• Realize you are doing the best you can as a parent. A child with a sibling who has mental illness is more likely to develop the following qualities: independent, dependable, compassionate and tolerant of others.

3. You and Your Spouse

My husband and I experienced guilt in the beginning after Ellie's first diagnosis sunk in. We may experience guilt for our mistakes and shortcomings, which can lead to experiencing discomfort. In order to feel more comfortable, we may begin blaming others. I would see my husband react to our daughter's behavior with outbursts toward her. It was hard for him to understand what she was feeling, and he had a difficult time seeing his child struggle without being able to fix the problem. I showed my guilt in sadness by crying alone in my room or in the bathroom. Families break apart because they have different ideas of how to parent or provide care for their children. It is important to make your relationship a priority and communicate.

We just celebrated our twenty-first anniversary at the time of writing this book. As I look over our marriage, I realize we had to overcome many challenges together. These experiences brought us closer together instead of tearing us apart. Our team is stronger than ever! The key is to learn how to manage the stress and challenges that are inevitable in marriage. Part of the adventure of marriage lies in facing difficulties together and growing more robust through the journey. Marriages aren't built on fairy tales. They're built on work. Married couples who experience true respect and understand that they need to work together as a team will find that genuine love grows stronger.

How to Protect Your Relationship

• Protect your partnership first, then come together to raise your sensitive child and additional children.

• Keep advice specific to the child. Don't place blame or guilt onto each other; this will tear you apart. Remember, you are partners and have made a commitment to each other.

• Respect is a big part of keeping your relationship together.

• Support each other. If one parent doesn't accept decisions or diagnoses, have discussions, find out the "why," and work through it together to find the best answer for your family.

• Spend quality time together without the children and don't talk about the challenges you are experiencing. Have fun together.

• If you have separated from your spouse, find a way to support each other for the sake of your child or children. It is tough enough to go through a crisis and then add in fighting with an ex. Find a way to support each other for the benefit of your child.

Tips for Couples

• Work on your relationship by finding time to be a couple. This could include dating, talking, and sharing. Carve out time for you to enjoy one another for a few hours weekly if possible. This helps build your resilience through tough times.

- Stay in communication. Send messages via text or email saying, "I love you," or "We got this," or check in to see how their day is going.

- Schedule a weekly check-in to sit together for fifteen minutes and talk about what is coming in the next week or what needs support.

- Give affirmations and thanks for even the most minor things.

- Spend some time apart. It is OK to spend time with friends or doing a hobby on your own. This gives you time to focus on yourself and come back feeling refreshed.

- It is OK to seek out counseling, whether individually or as a couple. This allows you to process your feelings in a healthy way when you're with your partner. You will receive perspective, balance, and guidance in a situation that can quickly become imbalanced.

4. Family as a Unit—Work Together or Against

It was Christmas break, when many families were together to celebrate, but ours had a different feel. There was a cloud of darkness surrounding our family due to our daughter leaving for the inpatient residential treatment facility. We hadn't told her, but I think she sensed that something was about to shake her world. I had presents wrapped under the tree. Ellie decided to rip open all her gifts and let me know she didn't like any of them. As my seven-year-old son stood watching and yelling for Ellie to stop, I tried to intervene, but she was determined to prove to me that she didn't receive any gifts that she wanted.

Even in moments like this, we stayed strong as a family. I made sure my son felt heard and supported by what he saw. Ellie returned to her room, her safe space. I knew I didn't do anything wrong and this was Ellie's way of trying to hurt me for all the hurt she was feeling. She eventually came out of her room and apologized for her behavior.

How to Work Together, Not Against Each Other

- The more resilient your family, the more you can handle problems without breaking apart. By showing perseverance and maintaining a sense of purpose, you can gain the resilience to overcome hardship and keep moving forward. Don't lose hope; hope is strong. Hope is the one thing stronger than fear, and no matter how bad things are, hope can help you see them through.

- Belief in each other. Families that are united provide meaningful support and encouragement to each other. There is an assumed, unspoken level of trust and commitment to one another.

- Sense of humor. Having a sense of humor during tense, troublesome moments can defuse the tension and has an immediate calming effect.

- Appreciation. Let your family members know you appreciate them. Strong families focus on the strengths of each other and not the faults.

- Commitment as a team. This creates excellent unity and trust within your family. The family shares a mission, values, and goals. The most important part of a team is trust and knowing that your family team will be there for you no matter what.

How to Come Together as a Team with Your Family

- Compromise. Come to a place of agreement. You must be willing to see things from another's perspective and work to find a middle ground.

- Express yourself. You need to feel you can be open with your feelings without judgment in a safe space.

- Respect. Listen to each other's thoughts. We don't always agree but it's important to be respectful and listen.

- Trust. When I would take our daughter to see different providers because I was following my intuition and what I felt was best for her, my spouse didn't question me because we had trust in each other. He saw how she shifted into a positive space.

- Positivity. The act of taking notice of your positive experiences is one of the most powerful ways to stay motivated and inspired. Even through the challenges, I found something positive. I was thankful we had access to care, that Ellie was still with us, and that we had a loving family. Whatever feels good to you, celebrate that. Remember that it's not the big things in life that count, it's the little ones. Like a sunny day, an unexpected compliment, or having your favorite snack available when you want it. Life requires both the big and the small.

5. You as an Individual

For Ellie and me, the most challenging times were centered around school. Yelling back and forth because she didn't want to go was a regular pattern. At one point I called my husband at work and said, "I can't do this anymore. I am not just Ellie's mom, I am also an employee, sister, daughter, friend, and wife." I left for work, and my husband came home and took Ellie to school. She listened to him, maybe in fear of his threats to take something away from her or out of pure exhaustion, but she got in the car with him and went to school. This gave him a chance to see what it was like to be me, as a mom to Ellie. Ellie consumed my life, and I forgot who I was. The feeling of losing yourself happens for many moms, especially when you have a child who takes over your life.

Once I started to work on my own healing journey, it changed the family. As moms, we are the heart-center of the family and can bring about a shift of change to our family members. This is a continuous journey of healing and learning. When you heal your past stories, forgive, discover your true self, and surround yourself by those that genuinely support you, you will find inner peace. I believe if I didn't start my transformation or awakening, we would be in the same space we were at the being of our story, navigating through mental illness. We all have the power within us to make a change. I didn't have a defined path as I started to work on my transformation. I felt divinely called or intuitively directed in the direction I needed to travel. So be open to the experience, however it may appear to you.

Self-love was the first tool I used in my journey back to me. I searched for the word "self-love" on the internet. I found the name Christine Arylo and a program she was teaching called the Path of Self-Love School. I immediately felt drawn to her and what she was offering. I registered for the twelve-month program, where I started to find peace with who I was and accept my true self. This is a continuous process of learning and unlearning.

SOCIAL LIFE

I was always in awe of Ellie when she stood at the church altar and read a scripture clearly and loudly at school mass with other students, faculty, and parents watching from the pews. I thought she was so brave, and I felt proud. Ellie was never nervous about reading in front of groups of people in her small elementary school, and she had many friends during her younger years with playdates, sleepovers, and birthday parties. Her social life changed as her mental illness became increasingly worse in her teen years. I think switching to a public school, teenage hormones, and mental illness created a perfect storm for chaos. Her life at the inpatient residential treatment facility forced her to socialize with others in her living space and school.

Ellie attended an online high school, which was an excellent option for her given her past experiences with school anxiety and fear of social situations with those she didn't know. While she thrived academically, what we found over those four years was that her social life declined. She went from being a social butterfly to being afraid to start a conversation with anyone.

Online schooling has its benefits and challenges. The online school created a safe environment for my daughter to receive an education but created a lack in peer interaction and social skills. My once very social child became an isolated teen.

Social life is so important for adolescents. To be with friends is perhaps hardwired in our brains. A child looks up to their family primarily to meet emotional needs, but they need independence, which is created when building a peer group of their choosing rather than family. When you lack friendships with your peers, you can feel lonely, guilty, or sad, or have a loss of interest in things that bring you pleasure.

Ellie's friends stopped coming around our house after she went to the inpatient residential treatment facility at fourteen. They moved on with their friendships and lives as teenagers. I was told that there were rumors at school that Ellie had died or moved away. Putting her back in that space didn't seem to be an option and is another reason we leaned toward online school. It gave her a safe environment at home and allowed her to focus on her education. I was frustrated that she had to give up the fun of attending football games, dances, and prom to feel safe learning. This doesn't seem right!

Ellie didn't have an interest in seeking out any social activities or making new friends when she was adjusting to her gifts as a sensitive empath and intuitive person. She did have two friends who were very understanding and supportive through everything, as well as a very tight-knit family that provided loving support.

How can we help our children be social?

- Be understanding. Don't push them into activities or friendships.

- Encourage them. Give them opportunities to be around other like-minded kids. If they enjoy robotics, see if there is a club in your community.

- Practice social skills. Social interactions are complex, and children don't always know how to behave or read cues from others. You can guide your child by role-playing or talking them through potential situations.

- Empathize. Validate their feelings.

- Sensitive people tend to have smaller groups of friends. We enjoy deeper conversations and not surface-level talks. It is OK if they have a small group of close friends.

BUILDING COMMUNITY

I didn't realize how important community was to my personal growth until I was a managing director of a local networking group for professional women. It turns out this experience brought more transformation and support than I ever expected.

In the beginning, I wasn't sharing the struggles we experienced with Ellie and her mental illness with many people, not even family. I did share more with my coworker Lori. She was someone I saw daily, and I felt safe sharing with her. It was comforting to have someone outside of my family listen to my daily stresses. When Ellie was eight years old and we received her first mental illness diagnosis, Lori was there to listen without judgment. I would chat with Lori daily and share updates with her on Ellie's progress and the challenges. I remember one conversation we had where she shared that one of her friends, who had a daughter with similar issues to Ellie, had to send their child away for treatment. When I heard that story, I thought, *Who would do that to their child, and how could it get that bad?* I even said, "I hope that never happens to us because I don't know what I would do." Well, it did happen to us about five years into the future. I worked at the YMCA, which already is a community, and over the years they supported me with my family life. They became part of my personal community, not just an employer. I took a leave of absence from my employment when Ellie was away for six months at the inpatient residential treatment facility. I felt it essential to focus on my family, and I knew Ellie would need me more than ever when she returned home.

When I brought Ellie to her weekly therapy appointments, I saw flyers pinned to the bulletin board and brochures laid out on the table for support groups, community support, resources, and discussion groups. I wouldn't even take a second glance. Nothing called out to me as a means of support for a parent to a child with mental illness. This doesn't mean these groups aren't beneficial to others. To me, a support group helps you cope, and provides an environment in which to talk about what you're going through and receive suggestions and resources.

I will openly share my challenges, but I don't seek out support outside of my inner circle. I have been this way most of my life. Any challenge I have gone through, I knew I could figure out with the support of those around me. I still say to my kids, "We will figure it out," even for the slightest problem.

I always knew there was a reason for our journey. The reason is you and others like you reading this book. I do think support groups and any variation are beneficial for people. I believe it is a personal choice and what works best for one person might not work for another.

What I do enjoy is being part of a community. To me, a community is a group of people who connect, empower, and support each other. When I was leading the community of women, I could be authentically me and feel accepted. This community was not about my child, yet it sparked change within me that moved us forward on our alternative journey with Ellie. I was able to be me and not a parent to a child with mental illness. I was a business owner, a supporting friend, a connector, a community builder, a working mom, a loving spouse, and a parent to two children.

It is important to find support or a sense of community in whatever form feels best to you.

Why a Support Group Would Be Helpful

- Connect with people who have experienced a similar situation because they understand the challenges.

- Receive and share resources. There are so many options that we don't know are available to us.

- A support group can be a safe place to share your story

with those who understand. This can feel powerful and you might be helping someone else.

• You feel less alone when others can relate to your situation.

Why a Community Would Be Helpful

• With community comes empowerment. When people feel empowered, they feel more confident and self-assured, enabling them to influence positive change.

• A community offers a space to meet a diverse group of people that become organically supportive.

• By connecting with someone, we create a bond. Because of this bond, we feel safe and secure enough to be ourselves, allowing us to be open and trusting.

• If you can't find an ideal community, I challenge you to create it. If you feel a need, I know there is someone else out in the universe with that similar need, and they would benefit from your support or community.

Chapter Eleven

FINDING YOUR VOICE

s I observe our family's journey to recognize the truth of who my daughter is as a sensitive, empath intuitive soul, I understand myself and past generations on a deeper level. We are deep thinkers and feelers, which can cause emotional distress if misunderstood by ourselves and others.

Being called shy, timid, and even stuck up throughout my younger years was because I didn't speak unless I had something important to say or felt comfortable with the people in my space. I was different from the others, so they labeled me with words that made sense to them. In turn, I carried those words as truth for much of my life.

As I worked through my self-love path, I also realized the importance of self-awareness and self-understanding. When you understand who you truly are in your soul and accept this to be true, you can begin to grow into your authentic self. Being your authentic self is being who you truly are as a person regardless of influence from others. Part of awakening is a deep understanding that you are not the person you thought you were.

Reflecting through my journey as a parent to Ellie, I can see that I struggled with self-acceptance, self-understanding, and self-awareness. My own struggles made it difficult for me to accept parts of my daughter. I didn't want her to be seen as different, so I pushed her into classes or groups with other kids, even at the expense of her own feelings or desires. I created an anxious child from my own inadequacy. Instead of embracing her differences and honoring her needs, I pushed her into what I thought society wanted from my child.

I came to a place of surrender when I could no longer control her. Ellie made this known by her extreme behavior, which was her way of letting me know I wasn't in control anymore. But this also led to the decision to send her to the inpatient residential treatment facility. This was needed to shake me awake to change myself and support her in a different direction.

Control is rooted in fear. I had so much fear—fear of being a bad parent, fear of losing my child, fear of my family breaking apart. When we trust that we're OK no matter what circumstances come our way, we let go and release control. This is surrendering. It takes courage to surrender.

I remember someone commenting to me that what I have experienced with Ellie takes courage. That comment didn't feel right to me. When I think of courage, I imagine someone running into a burning building to save another's life without thinking of their own life. I didn't have courage. I was doing what I thought was best for my child. Over many years I defied that word until one day, very recently, I read the definition—"mental or moral strength to venture, persevere, and withstand danger, fear, or difficulty"[17]—and realized, "Yes, I have courage."

Courage is what you have when you believe in yourself. It's an action we take, a decision we make.

Much of what I did to support Ellie took courage. I dealt with fear or difficulty, and persevered. Each appointment I took her to as we argued in the car, I knew I was doing what I had to do to help my child, just as I did with the trial and error of prescription medications in the hope of finding mood stability. The facilities where I left my child with people I didn't know, trusting that this would serve her best interest and find stability. Seeing my child strapped down on a gurney and put into the back of an ambulance to be taken to an inpatient hospitalization program for all family members' safety. The times I would open her bedroom door, not knowing if she was alive or dead because of her own choice. Dropping her off at an inpatient residential facility and walking out the door as tears ran down my cheeks, hoping this would be the final solution. And finally, listening to my own intuition and my child's, even if it was impractical by the standards of society and mainstream medicine. My courage led me to find my voice, be open to new perspectives, and trust my intuition.

I believe motherhood takes courage. It takes courage to bring a child into a world of unknown conditions. We support our children every day. We help our kids with their homework and make sure they get a good night's sleep before school. We even sit up with our children when they are sick. We listen to the experts about what our child should be doing at each milestone. We research the best tools and ideas to support our child. We learn we are so much stronger than we thought. We try to be our best selves and set a good example. We do what we must for our family without hesitation every day, and that might not feel courageous.

But I am here to tell you, it is!

When we find peace and balance, we create powerful shifts and far-reaching changes for generations that came before us and those coming after us. Generational healing is an act of courage. Speaking up will heal and make generational shifts.

I wanted to end the echo of cycles within my family's past. I wanted to stop hiding who we truly are as sensitive souls, which caused mental health struggles. Many families have generational trauma. We must begin to form new thoughts, traditions, and behaviors. This begins with taking action to enhance your personal healing. I am now setting an example for my children with my actions.

Ellie exemplified courage, and when and if she feels ready, she can take steps forward to continue down her own path.

It does take courage to trust oneself, to rely on one's instincts.

For so much of our lives, our inner voice and intuition were drowned out by authoritarian, parental messages, or perhaps by societal or cultural influences. If we really can pause, ponder, and listen to ourselves, our intuition can guide us through and maybe even give us wings.

SHIFTING SOCIETY'S PERSPECTIVE

When we go against the social norm in anything we do for ourselves or our family, we are courageous. The courage to speak up, the courage to ask questions, and the courage to take a different path should be honored, not dismissed.

You might think you cannot change the world canvas, but the fact is, you can. I know this truth from personal experience.

We can do this by speaking up and sharing our story—I hid my daughter's mental illness in the beginning. I was concerned of what others would think and if she would be accepted. By not being open, I was telling Ellie I didn't accept her, and I played into the stigma. When I shared our story openly with people in conversation, it was amazing how many others knew someone who was experiencing mental illness or had a child with mental illness. This led me to meet some amazing families with similar struggles, women I can call my friends who are also trying to make a difference in mental health.

Along the journey, I learned to speak up and share more. This took time and I started by sharing with safe family and friends. Expanding my voice to others in the arena of mental health, holistic care, and spirituality allowed me to embrace and trust my voice. I took courses in speaking on my topic, being focused on holistic care and mental health. I was once a young girl who was afraid to raise her hand in class because she did not want to be heard, and now I was speaking up and sharing my story. The story is more important than me and my fears of being seen.

Do not be afraid of having your voice heard or your words read. This shows there is a person behind the story, allowing for empathy. Share emotion. If you challenge someone's emotional attachment to a belief, you can move their support toward your perspective. Introduce evidence of what has worked or not worked for your family. The nurse from Ellie's doctor's office knew I was a safe person to ask about her medication. I was open about our experience, which allowed for her to share. Being open is a kind of invitation to others. What you share about yourself should encourage others to come in and contact you. To involve themselves with you. Being open can be difficult in the beginning. It makes us feel vulnerable. But it also is important in terms of really letting others get to understand what we are experiencing, and our beliefs.

THE FAMILY THAT SURVIVED

I believe many different conditions contributed to Ellie's anxiety and other mental illness diagnoses. It was not just one apparent factor, as it may have seemed with her original diagnosis. Now I can look back and see the different pieces that made the completed puzzle of Ellie's mental illness. Knowing that various factors were creating Ellie's anxiety and other mental health issues brought me acceptance that we did the best for her at the time with the knowledge and experience we had.

I don't blame anyone who was involved in support of Ellie's care over the years. All those working alongside us were doing what they believed was best for her at the time. What I do not agree with is how our medical system works when dealing with mental health. It feels very broken with a lack of resources, stigma, and limited access to quality care. We are starting to see more collaboration with holistic and alternative options. We need more than a one-size-fits-all approach. It did not work for Ellie, and I know she is not the only one that did not find success with this type of approach in the mental health system. Blame, shame, and guilt do not serve a positive purpose in healing. We chose acceptance as an essential way for building resilience.

Our intuition and strong advocacy need to play a part in the care of our children. When I listened inward to my intuition and Ellie's, along with finding the strength to speak up and question the direction of our life, we changed our journey. You can do the same!

We have *all* changed and shifted, and it feels like we have come full circle. All of you have experienced my healing journey with me, and I thank you for coming along for this ride. My challenging child has become a thriving twenty-one-year-old who has a fresh outlook on her future. She still has challenging days, but we have learned how to support her differently as a family. We are grateful for all the days we have together.

Our life is different than when we started our journey, but there are residual symptoms and continuous struggles. Awareness has allowed us to be supportive and open to conversations. In the beginning, we were lost and searching for answers as to why our beautiful daughter was aggressive, angry, defiant, and anxious. But we received a confirmation message from an Archangel that led us down a different path that felt in alignment and empowered us to make the best decisions for our child. This path used a holistic approach to her mental health. We learned about highly sensitive people and empaths. When not understood, we can be seen as a mental illness, but the way we see it is understanding our daughter as a spiritual, creative, intuitive empath. My awakening allowed me to trust our new path and elevate the family's vibration from sadness to a space of peace.

Ellie is a bright light seeking her way to shine in this world. Some days she does not want to participate in life and stays in her room, where she feels safe. Other days she wants to be out around others and taking part in life. It is still a day-to-day journey, and it probably always will be. We have told her that if she ever wants to go on prescription medication or seek therapy, we will support her in that decision. She continues to use her holistic options. Instead of therapy, she has Reiki; instead of prescription medications, she has flower essences, meditation, affirmations, crystals, essential oils, and Chinese herbs.

Since the beginning of our journey, we have had a solid and supportive family by our side. It brings such great joy to see my family all together. We have never been separated by arguments or disagreements. We are a resilient family with strong values. My heart is full when I hear my two children laughing together. Lucca is the funny guy in the house who loves to tell stories.

My husband and I have a typical marriage with ups and downs. But what keeps us together is the love and respect we have for each other. This has grown even stronger over time.

I share all of this with you because there is hope. If you are struggling, like we were, know that it can change. It takes work, but I believe in you.

As for me, I am more than a mom to a child with mental illness. My daughter inspired me and taught me so many lessons along our journey. And I know that she will continue to teach me in the years to come. I am an empowered parent to two amazing children, married to my supportive husband, Mario. I am a friend to many, a loving daughter, caring sister, and healer with my message. Thank you for allowing me to share my message and journey to understanding and healing with you. I hope it brings you some awareness to look at things differently, feel empowered in your choices, and listen inward to your own wisdom and that of your child. Know that you, too, have a voice, a story, and a message. Embrace it because it is who you are.

FURTHER RESOURCES

You Can Heal Your Life by Louise Hay

The Highly Sensitive Person: How to Thrive When the World Overwhelms You by Elaine N. Aron, PhD

The Highly Sensitive Child: Helping our Children Thrive When the World Overwhelms Them by Elaine N. Aron, PhD

The Empath's Survival Guide: Life Strategies for Sensitive People by Judith Orloff

Worthy: Boost Your Self-Worth to Grow Your Net Worth by Nancy Levin

Madly in Love with ME: The Daring Adventure of Becoming Your Own Best Friend by Christine Arylo

Reform Your Inner Mean Girl: 7 Steps to Stop Bullying Yourself and Start Loving Yourself by Christine Arylo

The Universe Has Your Back: Transform Fear to Faith by Gabrielle Bernstein

Theta Healing: Introducing an Extraordinary Energy-Healing Modality by Vianna Stibal

The Strength of Sensitivity: Understanding Empathy for a Life of Emotional Peace & Balance by Kyra Mesich, PsyD

The Secret Language of Your Body by Inna Segal

It Didn't Start with You: How Inherited Family Trauma Shapes Who We Are and How to End the Cycle by Mark Wolynn

Bliss and Blessings: the Divine Alchemy of the Star Flower and Gemstone Essences by Star Riparetti

The Children of Now . . . Evolution: How We Can Support the Fast-Forward Evolution of Our Children and Our Race by Meg Blackburn Losy, PhD

The Higly Intuitive Child: A Guide to Understanding and Parenting Unusually Sensitive and Empathic Children by Catherine Crawford

Becoming an Empowered Empath: How to Clear Energy, Set Boundaries & Embody Your Intuition by Wendy De Rosa

Love Warrior: A Memoir by Glennon Doyle

I Think, I Am!: Teaching Kids the Power of Affirmations by Louise L. Hay and Kristina Tracy

Just As You Are by Jen Harrison

The Emerging Sensitive: A Guide for Finding Your Place in the World by Maria Hill

The Healed Empath: The Highly Sensitive Person's Guide to Transforming Trauma and Anxiety, Trusting Your Intuition, and Moving from Overwhelm to Empowerment by Kristen Schwartz

ABOUT THE AUTHOR

Heather Nardi is the author of four collaborative books, including three Amazon bestsellers. Her writing has appeared on *Thrive Global, Elephant Journal, The Highly Sensitive Refuge*, and *Medium*. Heather dedicates her career to supporting highly sensitive and empathic moms in living healthy, empowered lives. She draws from her extensive education as a holistic life coach and spiritual practitioner to create specialized tools and programs for sensitive mothers. Born and raised in Minnesota, Heather spends her downtime with her kids and spouse, usually out in nature or watching a movie.

NOTES

1   "Gad-7 (General Anxiety Disorder-7)," Official website of the U.S. Health Resources & Services Administration, August 2, 2019, https://www.hrsa.gov/behavioral-health/gad-7-general-anxiety-disorder-7.

2   Elayne Daniels, "Highly Sensitive People," Dr. Elayne Daniels Psychotherapy & Consultation, March 3, 2021, https://www.drelaynedaniels.com/the-highly-sensitive-person/.

3   Judith Orloff, MD, "4 Reasons Why People Become Empaths: From Trauma to Genetics," Dr. Judith Orloff, September 8, 2021, https://drjudithorloff.com/4-reasons-why-people-become-empaths-from-trauma-to-genetics/.

4   Maureen Gaspari, "Highly Sensitive or Sensory Processing Disorder?" The Highly Sensitive Child, April 2, 2019, https://www.thehighlysensitivechild.com/highly-sensitive-or-sensory-processing-disorder/.

5   Lisa Natcharian, "Why Are So Many Gifted Children Also Highly Sensitive?" Institute for Educational Advancement, April 18, 2017, https://educationaladvancement.org/blog-many-gifted-children-also-highly-sensitive/.

6   Sadiya Qamar (Contributor), "Highly Sensitive Child—Signs, Habits & Parenting," MomJunction, June 8, 2021, https://www.momjunction.com/articles/parenting-tips-to-handle-a-highly-sensitive-child_00336867/.

7   "Help for Emotionally Hypersensitive Children on the Autism Spectrum," My Aspergers Child, accessed October 8, 2021, https://www.myaspergerschild.com/2015/06/help-for-emotionally-hypersensitive.html.

8   Judith Orloff, MD, "The Difference between Empaths and Highly Sensitive People," Dr. Judith Orloff, May 21, 2021, https://drjudithorloff.com/the-difference-between-empaths-and-highly-sensitive-people/.

9   Rebecca Rosen, "What Is a Medium?" Oprah, May 26, 2010, https://www.oprah.com/spirit/what-is-a-medium-rebecca-rosen.

10   Ibid.

11   "The Highly Sensitive Child," Psychology Today, Sussex Publishers, accessed October 8, 2021, https://www.psychologytoday.com/us/blog/creative-development/201106/the-highly-sensitive-child.

12   "Learn How to Speak Up for Your Child," Kiwi Families, October 18, 2016, https://www.kiwifamilies.co.nz/learn-how-to-speak-up-for-your-child/.

13   "March Newsletter," Brighton Area Schools, accessed October 8, 2021, https://www.brightonk12.com/cms/lib/MI02209968/Centricity/Domain/27/March2019Newsletter.pdf.

14   Judith Orloff, "The Empathic Eater," in *The Empath's Survival Guide: Life Strategies for Sensitive People* (Sounds True, Inc., 2018).

15   William Lee Rand, "Reiki in Hospitals," Reiki, July 12, 2019, retrieved October 8, 2021, https://www.reiki.org/articles/reiki-hospitals.

16   "Aromatherapy: Why Essential Oils Are Being Used in Hospitals," Pierre Fabre, June 8, 2016, retrieved October 8, 2021, https://www.pierre-fabre.com/en-us/news/aromatherapy-why-essential-oils-are-being-used-in-hospitals.

17   Merriam-Webster, "Courage," Merriam-Webster, retrieved October 9, 2021, https://www.merriam-webster.com/dictionary/courage.